Traction and
Orthopaedic Appliances

To
E.G.S.

Traction and Orthopaedic Appliances

JOHN D.M. STEWART

MA (Cantab), FRCS (England)
Consultant Orthopaedic Surgeon,
Chichester, and Worthing District
Groups of Hospitals

JEFFREY P. HALLETT

MA (Oxon), FRCS (England)
Consultant Orthopaedic Surgeon,
The Ipswich Hospitals

SECOND EDITION

CHURCHILL LIVINGSTONE
EDINBURGH LONDON MELBOURNE AND NEW YORK 1983

CHURCHILL LIVINGSTONE
Medical Division of Longman Group Limited

Distributed in the United States of America by
Churchill Livingstone Inc., 1560 Broadway, New York,
N.Y. 10036, and by associated companies,
branches and representatives throughout the world.

First edition 1975
Second edition 1983
  Reprinted 1985
ISBN 0 443 02004 3

British Library Cataloguing in Publication Data
Stewart, John D.M.
  Traction and orthopaedic appliances.—2nd ed
  1. Orthopedic apparatus
  I. Title   II. Hallett, Jeffrey P.
  617'307   RD755

Library of Congress Cataloging in Publication Data
Stewart, John D.M.
  Traction and orthopaedic appliances.
  Includes bibliographies and index.
  1. Orthopedic traction. 2. Orthopedic
apparatus. I. Hallett, Jeffrey P.
II. Title. [DNLM: 1. Orthopedic equipment.
2. Traction. WE 26 S849t]
RD736.T7S73 1983 617'.3 82-9632

Produced by Longman Group (FE) Ltd
Printed in Hong Kong

Preface to
the Second Edition

This book is still intended for the use of junior doctors and the other staff of orthopaedic and trauma wards and clinics, who are concerned in the day to day management of patients.

The new techniques which have become popular in the treatment of fractures, traction in the management of fractures of the upper limb, the prescription of orthoses and the new terminology used in their description, as well as the many new casting materials which have been developed, have been described. In addition the previous chapters on *Management of Patients in Traction* and *Tourniquets* have been completely rewritten.

We wish to thank the many people who have assisted us in the preparation of this edition, in particular Mr G. L. W. Bonney for his help with the chapter on *Tourniquets*; Miss J. Thomas and Mrs A. Stickland for their instructive criticism of the chapter on *Management of Patients in Traction*; Mr J. Florence for his assistance with the unravelling of the tangled web of orthotic terminology and the prescription of orthoses; Mr P. Shaw for showing us how surgical footwear is made; and finally the many manufacturers and distributors of the splinting and casting materials discussed in Chapter 13.

Bognor Regis, 1983
J.D.M.S.
J.P.H.

Preface to
the First Edition

This book is written primarily for the use of orthopaedic house surgeons and junior registrars, and of the nursing and physiotherapy staff of accident and orthopaedic wards.

Many of the procedures and appliances described here are in common usage. The details, however, of how to carry out these procedures, their contra-indications and complications, and how to check the various applicances, are not available in the standard textbooks. This book is intended to rectify this omission and to be a practical source of instruction in these matters.

I wish to thank the many people who have assisted me in the preparation of this book, in particular Mr W. H. Tuck, without whose considerable guidance the chapters on *Spinal Supports, Lower Limb Bracing* and *Footwear* would have been incomplete; Dr J. D. G. Troup for his help with the section on the biomechanics of the spine; Mr F. G. St C. Strange and Mr G. R. Fisk who have kindly helped me in the description of their methods of applying traction to the lower limb; and to the staff of the Physiotherapy Department of the Royal National Orthopaedic Hospital for their assistance with the chapters on Walking Aids and Crutch Walking. I also wish to express my gratitude to Professor R. G. Burwell who advised me on the original script, to Mr J. Crawford Adams who read the final draft, and to Dr R. R. Mason for his careful reading of the proofs.

Bognor Regis, 1974   J.D.M.S.

Contents

Contents

1.

Traction

When a limb is painful as a result of inflammation of a joint or a fracture of one of the bones, the controlling muscles go into spasm. The antagonistic muscles in a limb are not all equally powerful, with the result that when muscle spasm is present, the action of the more powerful muscles can produce a deformity which may seriously impair the future function of the limb.

Inflammation of the hip joint commonly results in a flexion, adduction and lateral rotation deformity, the presence of which causes *apparent shortening* of the affected lower limb.

When the shaft of the femur is fractured at the junction of the upper and middle thirds, the proximal fragment is flexed and abducted by the pull of the ilio-psoas and hip abductor muscles respectively, and the distal fragment is adducted by the adductor muscles of the thigh. In addition, if apposition of the fragments is lost, marked shortening of the femur occurs.

Traction, when applied to an injured limb, can overcome the effect of the original deforming force, and thus can be used to reduce a fracture or a dislocation of a joint (sliding traction — see Ch. 4). In addition by overcoming muscle spasm and, in certain traction systems, the effect of gravity, traction can relieve pain and allow the limb to be rested in the best functional position. Traction also controls movement of an injured part of the body and thus aids in the healing of bone and soft tissues.

METHODS OF APPLYING TRACTION

To apply traction, a satisfactory grip must be obtained on a part of the body. In the case of a limb, the traction force may be applied through the skin — *skin traction* — or via the bones — *skeletal traction.*

A traction force may be applied also to other parts of the body. Pelvic traction is described in Chapter 4, and spinal traction in Chapter 6.

SKIN TRACTION

The traction force is applied over a large area of skin. This spreads the load, and is more comfortable and efficient. In the treatment of fractures, the traction force must be applied only to the limb distal to the fracture site, otherwise the efficiency of the traction force is reduced.

The maximum traction weight which can be applied with skin traction is 15lb (6.7kg).

Two methods of applying skin traction are commonly used.

Adhesive skin traction

Adhesive strapping which can be stretched only transversely is used. The necessary apparatus can be assembled individually, but prepared skin traction kits for use in adults or children can be obtained commercially.

Elastoplast Skin Traction Kits* are available from Smith and Nephew Ltd. Some patients are allergic to adhesive strapping. For these patients other preparations which do not utilize an adhesive containing zinc oxide can be used, for example Tractac* (Johnson & Johnson Ltd) which uses an acrylic adhesive and Seton Skin Traction Kit* (Seton Products Ltd). Two other preparations to which allergic reactions have not been reported are Orthotrac* (OEC Orthopaedic Ltd) and Skin-Trac* (Zimmer, USA).

APPLICATION OF ADHESIVE STRAPPING

— Shave the limb (shaving is not required with Tractac, Orthotrac and Skin-Trac).
— Protect the malleoli/ulnar head and radial styloid process from friction with a strip of felt, foam rubber or a few turns of a crepe or elasticated bandage under the strapping.
— Starting at the ankle/wrist, but leaving a loop projecting 2 inches (5.0 cm) beyond the distal end of the limb to allow free movement of the foot/fingers, apply the widest possible strapping to each side of the limb.
Lower limb. The strapping is applied to the lateral and medial aspects of the limb. On the lateral aspect the strapping must lie slightly behind and parallel to a line between the lateral malleolus and the greater trochanter. On the medial aspect the strapping must lie slightly in front of the above line to encourage medial rotation of the limb (Fig. 1.1).

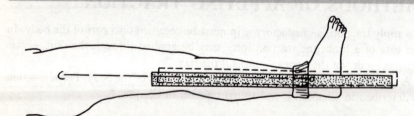

Fig. 1.1 Skin traction: note that on the lateral side, the strapping lies slightly behind and parallel to a line between the lateral malleolus and the greater trochanter.

*See Appendix

— Avoid wrinkles and creases. If necessary, nick the strapping to ensure that it lies flat.

— Avoid bony prominences — malleoli, tibial crest, patella, ulnar head, radial styloid process, humeral epicondyles.

— Apply a crepe or elasticated bandage firmly over the strapping starting at the ankle/wrist, and continuing up the limb (Fig. 1.2). The bandage must not be applied tightly around the limb. A tight bandage may cause skin and vascular complications.

— Check that a spreader and traction cords are present.

— Attach the required traction weight.

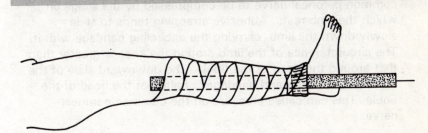

Fig. 1.2 Skin traction.

Non-adhesive skin traction

Ventfoam Skin Traction Bandage* (The Scholl Manufacturing Co. Ltd) consists of lengths of soft, ventilated latex foam rubber laminated to a strong cloth backing. Other non-adhesive skin traction systems are Specialist Foam Traction* (Johnson & Johnson Ltd) and Notac Traction* (Seton Products Ltd). These are useful on thin and atrophic skin, or when there is sensitivity to adhesive strapping. They are applied in the same way as adhesive strapping, but as their grip is less than that of adhesive strapping, frequent reapplications may be necessary. The traction weight used should not exceed 10lb (4.5kg).

CONTRAINDICATIONS TO SKIN TRACTION

1. Abrasions of the skin
2. Lacerations of the skin in the area to which the traction is to be applied
3. Impairment of circulation — varicose ulcers, impending gangrene
4. Dermatitis
5. Marked shortening of the bony fragments, when the traction weight required will be greater than can be applied through the skin.

*See Appendix

COMPLICATIONS OF SKIN TRACTION

1. Allergic reactions to the adhesive.
2. Excoriation of the skin from slipping of the adhesive strapping.
3. Pressure sores around the malleoli and over the tendo calcaneus.
4. Common peroneal nerve palsy. This may result from two causes.
   Rotation of the limb is difficult to control with skin traction. There is a tendency for the limb to rotate laterally and for the common peroneal nerve to be compressed by the slings on which the limb rests. Adhesive strapping tends to slide slowly down the limb, carrying the encircling bandage with it. The circumference of the limb around the knee is greater than that around the head of the fibula. The downward slide of the adhesive strapping and bandage is halted at the head of the fibula. This can cause pressure on the common peroneal nerve.

SKELETAL TRACTION

For skeletal traction, a metal pin or wire is driven through the bone. By this means the traction force is applied directly to the skeleton (for spinal traction, see Ch. 6).

Skeletal traction is seldom necessary in the management of upper limb fractures. It is used frequently in the management of lower limb fractures. It may be employed as a means of reducing or of maintaining the reduction of a fracture. It should be reserved for those cases in which skin traction is contraindicated. A serious complication of skeletal traction is osteomyelitis.

Steinmann pin

Steinmann pins (Steinmann, 1916) are rigid stainless steel pins of varying lengths, 4 to 6 millimetres in diameter. After insertion, a special stirrup (Böhler, 1929), illustrated in Figure 1.3, is attached to the pin. The *Böhler stirrup* allows the direction of the traction to be varied without turning the pin in the bone.

Denham pin

The Denham pin (Denham, 1972) illustrated in Figure 1.4 is identical to a Steinmann pin except for a short raised threaded length situated towards the end held in the introducer. This threaded portion engages the bony cortex and reduces the risk of the pin sliding. This type of pin is particularly suitable for use in cancellous bone, such as the calcaneus, or in osteoporotic bone.

Kirschner wire

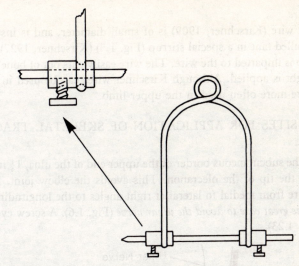

Fig. 1.3 Böhler stirrup with Steinmann pin.

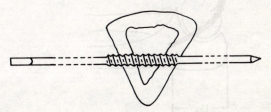

Fig. 1.4 Denham pin.

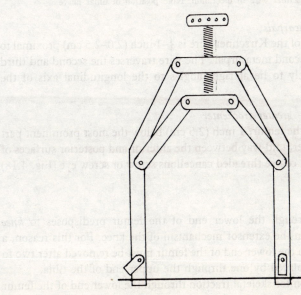

Fig. 1.5 Kirschner wire strainer.

Kirschner wire

A Kirschner wire (Kirschner, 1909) is of small diameter, and is insufficiently rigid until pulled taut in a special stirrup (Fig. 1.5) (Kirschner, 1927). Rotation of the stirrup is imparted to the wire. The wire easily cuts out of bone if a heavy traction weight is applied. Although Kirschner wires can be used in the lower limb, they are more often used in the upper limb.

COMMON SITES FOR APPLICATION OF SKELETAL TRACTION

Olecranon

Just deep to the subcutaneous border of the upper end of the ulna, $1\frac{1}{4}$ inches (3.0 cm) distal to the tip of the olecranon. This avoids the elbow joint. Drive the Kirschner wire from medial to lateral at right angles to the longitudinal axis of the ulna. *Take great care to avoid the ulnar nerve* (Fig. 1.6). A screw eye also can be used (Fig. 4.23).

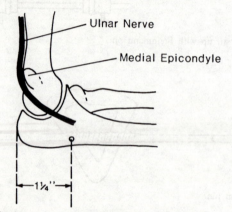

Ulnar Nerve

Medial Epicondyle

1¼"

Fig. 1.6 Position for Kirschner wire in olecranon. Note position of ulnar nerve.

Second and third metacarpals

The point of insertion of the Kirschner wire is $\frac{3}{4}$–1 inch (2.0–2.5 cm) proximal to the distal end of the second metacarpal. The wire traverses the second and third metacarpals transversely to lie at right angles to the longitudinal axis of the radius (Fig. 1.7).

Upper end of femur — greater trochenter

The lateral surface of the femur, 1 inch (2.5 cm) below the most prominent part of the greater trochanter, mid-way between the anterior and posterior surfaces of the femur (Fig. 1.8). A coarse threaded cancellous screw or screw eye (Fig. 4.18) is used (see Ch. 4).

Lower end of femur

Prolonged traction through the lower end of the femur predisposes to *knee stiffness* from fibrosis in the extensor mechanism of the knee. For this reason, a Steinmann pin through the lower end of the femur must be removed after two to three weeks and be replaced by one through the upper end of the tibia.

The point of insertion for skeletal traction through the lower end of the femur can be determined in two ways.

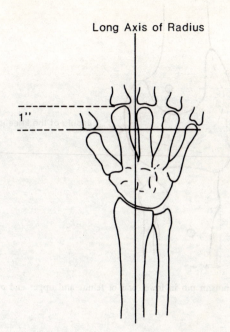

Fig. 1.7 Position for Kirschner wire in second and third metacarpals. Note that the wire is at right angles to the long axis of the radius.

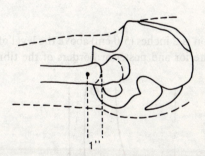

Fig. 1.8 Position for screw eye in upper end of femur for lateral femoral traction.

1. Draw a line from before backwards at the level of the upper pole of the patella. Draw a second line from below upwards anterior to the head of the fibula. Where these two lines intersect is the point of insertion of a Steinmann pin (Fig. 1.9).

2. Just proximal to the upper limit of the lateral femoral condyle. In the average adult this point is $1\frac{1}{4}$ inches (3.0 cm) proximal to the articulation between the lateral femoral condyle and the lateral tibial plateau.

Care must be taken to avoid entering the knee joint. The lateral fold of the capsule of the knee joint reaches $\frac{1}{2}$ to $\frac{3}{4}$ inch (1.25–2.0 cm) above the level of the joint (Fig. 1.9).

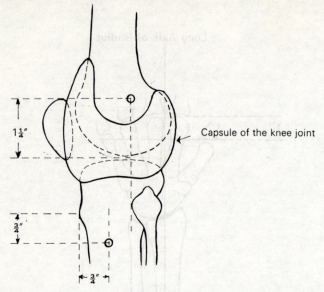

Fig. 1.9 Position for Steinmann pin in lower end of femur and upper end of tibia.

Upper end of tibia
The point of insertion is $\frac{3}{4}$ inch (2.0 cm) behind the crest, just below the level of the tubercle of the tibia (Fig. 1.9). The pin should be driven from the lateral to the medial side of the limb to avoid damage to the common peroneal nerve.

Lower end of tibia
The point of insertion is 2 inches (5.0 cm) above the level of the ankle joint, midway between the anterior and posterior borders of the tibia (Fig. 1.10).

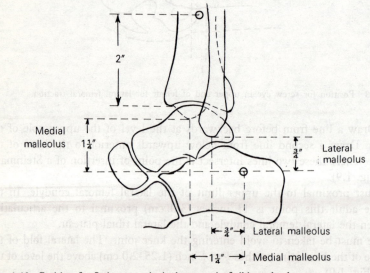

Fig. 1.10 Position for Steinmann pin in lower end of tibia and calcaneus.

Calcaneus

The point of insertion is $\frac{3}{4}$ inch (2.0 cm) below and behind the lateral malleolus. (As the lateral malleolus lies $\frac{1}{2}$ inch (1.25 cm) more posterior and distal than the medial malleolus, the above point corresponds with that $1\frac{1}{4}$ inches (3.0 cm) below and behind the medial malleolus. Care must be taken to avoid entering the subtalar joint (Fig. 1.10).

The insertion of a Steinmann pin through the calcaneus may result in stiffness of the subtalar joint, or more seriously, in infection in the bone. However, with a pin in this site, the traction force is applied in the line of the calf muscles, counteracts their pull, and thereby reduces the deforming action of these muscles on the fracture. When possible the lower tibial site for insertion of a Steinmann pin should be used.

APPLICATION OF SKELETAL TRACTION INSERTION OF STEINMANN PIN — LOWER LIMB

- Use general or local anaesthesia. If local anaesthesia is used, the skin and the periosteum on both sides of the limb must be infiltrated.
- Shave the skin.
- Use full aseptic precautions — mask, cap, gown, gloves and drapes.
- Paint the skin with iodine and spirit.
- Drape skin towels under and around the limb.
- Mount the Steinmann pin on the introducer.
- Ask an assistant to hold the limb in the same degree of lateral rotation as the normal limb (Fig. 1.11) and with the ankle at a right angle. This ensures that if the limb is resting upon a pillow, the outer (lateral) end of the Steinmann pin does not press on either the pillow or mattress thus tending to cause a medial rotational deformity at the fracture site.
- Identify the site of insertion (see above).

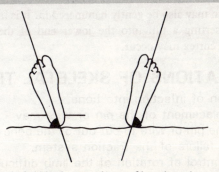

Fig. 1.11 The limb must be held in the same degree of lateral rotation as the normal limb; the Steinmann pin lies horizontally.

- Hold the pin horizontally and at right angles to the long axis of the limb (Fig. 1.12).
- Drive the pin from lateral to medial, through the skin and the bone with a gentle twisting motion of the forearm, while keeping the flexed elbow against the side of your body, and taking care to avoid putting your other hand opposite the site where the pin will emerge.
- Apply on each side a small cotton wool pad, soaked in Tinct. Benzoin, around the pin to seal the wounds. Always use two separate pads. One strip of gauze wound back and forth across the shin and around the Steinmann pin may cause a pressure sore. Tinct. Benzoin is the best sealing compound as it will stick to skin and metal.
- Fit the Böhler stirrup.
- Apply guards over the ends of the pin.

Longitudinal Axis of Limb

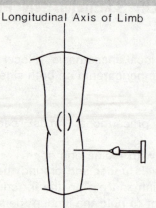

Fig. 1.12   The Steinmann pin is inserted at right angles to the longitudinal axis of the limb.

By not incising the skin with a scalpel prior to inserting the Steinmann pin by hand, a much tighter fit around the pin is obtained. If the Steinmann pin is inserted with a power drill the skin must be incised first. The skin must not be puckered. If the skin does pucker, it must be incised and one or two sutures inserted if necessary.

A Steinmann pin may also be gently hammered in. It is inadvisable to use this method when inserting a pin into the lower end of the femur or tibia, as splintering of the cortex may occur.

COMPLICATIONS OF SKELETAL TRACTION

1. Introduction of infection into bone.
2. Incorrect placement of the pin or wire may
   - Allow the pin or wire to cut out of the bone causing pain and the failure of the traction system.
   - Make control of rotation of the limb difficult.
   - Make the application of splints difficult.

— Result in an uneven pull being applied to the ends of the pin or wire and thus cause the pin or wire to move in the bone. This movement will result in an increased risk of infection in the bone and ischaemic necrosis of the skin around the pin or wire from pressure on the skin by the Böhler stirrup or Kirschner wire strainer.

3. Distraction at the fracture site as very large traction forces can be applied through skeletal traction.
4. Ligamentous damage if a large traction force is applied through a joint for a prolonged period of time.
5. Damage to epiphyseal growth plates when used in children. Genu recurvatum can occur as a late complication of the treatment of a fracture of the femoral shaft in children with traction through the upper end of the tibia (Bjerkreim and Benum, 1975; Van Meter and Branick, 1980).
6. Depressed scars. These can be prevented if the pin track is pinched at the time of removal of the pin, to rupture the bridge of fibrous tissue which forms between the skin and periosteum (Douglas et al, 1980).

COUNTER-TRACTION

One of the reasons for applying a traction force to a part of the body is to counteract the deforming effects of *muscle spasm*. The muscles in spasm tend to draw the distal part of the body in a proximal direction. A traction force applied to the affected part of the body will overcome *muscle spasm* only if another force acting in the opposite direction — *counter-traction* — is applied at the same time as the traction force. If counter-traction is not applied, the whole body will tend to be pulled in the direction of the traction force, and muscle spasm will not be overcome.

FIXED TRACTION

One method of obtaining counter-traction is by applying a force against a fixed point on the body, proximal to the attachments of the muscles in spasm. A similar situation exists when an attempt is made to extract a cork from a bottle. The neck of the bottle is gripped in one hand and the corkscrew in the other. When a traction force is *initially* applied to the corkscrew, another force, acting in the opposite direction (counter-traction), is applied at the same time to the bottle, the *counter-traction force* passing along the arm to the neck of the bottle. This mechanical arrangement is called *fixed traction*.

To apply a force against a fixed point on the body, an appliance, for example a Thomas's splint (see Ch. 2) is used. The ring of the splint snugly encircles the root of the limb. The traction cords are tied to the distal end of the splint, and the counter-traction force passes along the side bars of the splint to the ring and hence to the body proximal to the attachment of the muscles in spasm (Fig. 3.1).

Fixed traction is discussed in Chapter 3.

SLIDING TRACTION

Gravity may be utilized to provide *counter-traction* by tilting the bed so that the patient tends to slide in the opposite direction to that of the traction force. This is called *sliding traction* and is discussed in Chapter 4. A splint is often used when sliding traction is employed, but the function of the splint in this instance is merely to cradle the limb.

REFERENCES

Bjerkreim, I. & Benum, P. (1975) Genu recurvatum. A late complication of tibial wire traction in fractures of the femur in children. *Acta Orthopaedica Scandinavica*, **46**, 1012.
Böhler, L. (1929) *The Treatment of Fractures*. English translation by Steinberg, M.E., p. 38 and p. 39, Fig. 56. Vienna: Maudrich.
Denham, R. A. (1972) Personal communication.
Douglas, G., Rang, M. & Clements, N. (1980) The prevention of depressed scars after the use of skeletal traction. *Journal of Bone and Joint Surgery*, **62-A**, 307.
Kirschner, M. von (1909) Ueber Nagelextension. *Beiträge zur Klinischen Chirurgie*, **64**, 266.
Kirschner, M. von (1927) Verbesserungen Der Drahtextension. *Archiv Für Klinische Chirurgie*, **148**, 651.
Steinmann, F. von (1916) Die Nagelextension. *Ergebnisse Der Chirurgie und Orthopädie*, **9**, 520.
Van Meter, J.W. & Branick, R.I. (1980) Bilateral genu recurvatum after skeletal traction: a case report. *Journal of Bone and Joint Surgery*, **62-A**, 837.

2.

The Thomas's and Fisk splints

THOMAS'S SPLINT

The splint which today is called the Thomas's splint was described originally by Hugh Owen Thomas (Thomas, 1876) as a knee appliance which he used in the ambulant management of chronic or subacute inflammation of the knee joint. The present splint consists of a padded oval metal ring covered with soft leather, to which are attached inner and outer side bars. These side bars which exactly bisect the oval ring, are of unequal length so that the padded ring is set at an angle of 120 degrees to the inner side bar. At the distal end the two side bars are joined together in the form of a 'W'. The outer side bar is often angled out 2 inches (5.0 cm) below the padded ring, to clear a prominent greater trochanter (Fig. 3.1).

The padded ring is made in different sizes and the side bars in varying lengths.

CHOOSING A THOMAS'S SPLINT

1. **Measure the oblique circumference of the thigh immediately below the gluteal fold and ischial tuberosity.** The line of measurement is oblique and must correspond with the inclination of the ring of the splint (Fig. 2.1). This measurement equals the *internal* circumference of the padded ring. If the above measurement cannot be taken without causing the patient pain, measure the oblique circumference of the normal thigh. Add 2 inches (5.0 cm) to this measurement if there is much swelling of the injured thigh. Accuracy is required if fixed traction is intended. With sliding traction, accuracy is not so important because the function of the splint is merely to support the limb.

2. **Measure the distance from the crotch to the heel** *and add 6 to 9 inches (15 to 23 cm).* This distance equals the length of the inner side bar (Fig. 2.1).

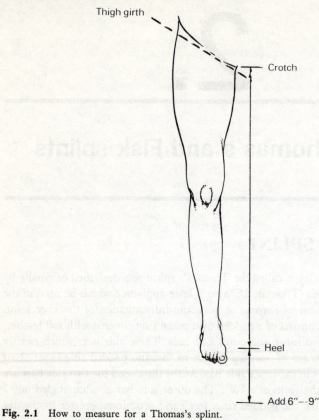

Fig. 2.1 How to measure for a Thomas's splint.

PREPARING A THOMAS'S SPLINT

1. Fashion slings, between the side bars, on which the limb can rest.
Cut an adequate length of 6 inch (15.0 cm) wide domette bandage or calico. It is better to cut off excess length later, than to have to change a sling which is too short, after the limb has been placed in the splint.
Pass the length of domette bandage or calico around the inner side bar. Then pass *both ends above* the outer side bar (Fig. 2.2).

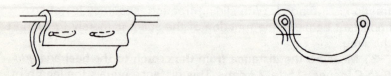

Fig. 2.2 Detail of fixing of sling to inner and outer side bars of a Thomas's splint.

Fasten the two ends to the sling so formed with two large safety pins or toothed clips.

In this way the tension of the sling can be adjusted easily after the splint has been fitted to the limb (Fig. 2.2), to ensure uniform support of the limb, and to avoid excess pressure in the region of the neck of the fibula and the tendo calcaneus.

The *proximal sling* leaves a triangular area of thigh unsupported because of the obliquity of the ring of the splint with the side bars. This triangular area can be supported by passing the length of domette bandage around the ring of the splint as well as the side bars (Fig. 2.3) (Strange, 1965).

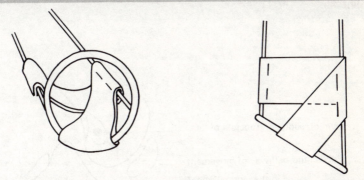

Fig. 2.3 Method of arranging the proximal sling to obliterate the triangular gap which results from the obliquity of the ring of a Thomas's splint.

The *distal sling* must end $2\frac{1}{2}$ inches (6.0 cm) above the heel to avoid pressure sores developing over the tendo calcaneus (Fig. 2.4).

The slings tend to slip distally on the side bars of the Thomas's splint. This can be prevented by pinning each sling to the one above or by binding the side bars with zinc oxide strapping before applying the slings.

2. Line the slings with Gamgee tissue.

3. Fashion one large pad from Gamgee tissue or cotton wool. This pad should measure roughly 6 by 9 inches (15 by 23 cm) and be about 2 inches (5.0 cm) thick when compressed. Place this pad transversely under the lower part of the thigh to maintain the normal anterior bowing of the femoral shaft (Fig. 2.4).

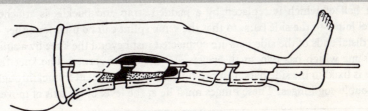

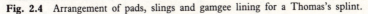

Fig. 2.4 Arrangement of pads, slings and gamgee lining for a Thomas's splint.

4. If the leg is to be supported in a knee-flexion piece, the hinge must coincide with the axis of movement of the knee joint. The movement of flexion and extension at a normal knee joint is not one of simple hinge movement, but is complex, following a polycentric pathway (the instant centres determined for each increment of flexion moving posteriorly in a spiral pattern (Gunston, 1971), as shown in Fig. 2.5).

However, from the point of view of the siting of the hinge of a knee-flexion piece, the axis of movement is taken to lie level with the adductor tubercle of the femur (Fig. 2.5).

5. After the splint has been fitted, bandage the limb into the splint.

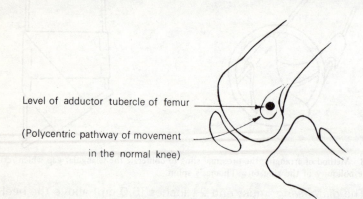

Level of adductor tubercle of femur

(Polycentric pathway of movement in the normal knee)

Fig. 2.5 Hinge of knee-flexion piece is sited level with the adductor tubercle of the femur.

FISK SPLINT

The splint described by Fisk (1944) consists of a modified Thomas's splint to which a knee-flexion piece is attached. The Thomas's splint is modified by removing the side bars beyond the level of the knee joint, and turning the cut ends of the side bars horizontally outwards to form small rings. A knee-flexion piece is fixed firmly to the side bars just proximal to these rings, level with the axis of movement of the knee joint.

The splint is now purpose-designed* (Fig. 2.6). The padded groin ring, the front half of which is replaced by a padded strap and buckle, is attached by swivel joints to the side bars, so that the same splint can be used for either limb. The distal ends of the side bars are connected just beyond the knee by a squared-off frame which has two small eyelets at each upper corner. The knee-flexion piece is fixed to the side bars, just proximal to the squared-off frame, through off-set double-cog hinges. These hinges must lie at the level of the axis of movement

*See Appendix.

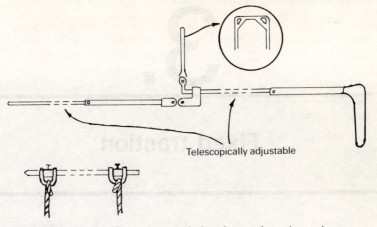

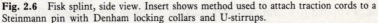

Telescopically adjustable

Fig. 2.6 Fisk splint, side view. Insert shows method used to attach traction cords to a Steinmann pin with Denham locking collars and U-stirrups.

of the knee joint when the splint is applied to the limb. The side bars of the thigh and knee-flexion parts of the splint are adjustable telescopically, thus enabling all lengths of lower limb to be accommodated.

Application of sliding traction with the Fisk splint is described in Chapter 4, and suspension of the splint in Chapter 5.

REFERENCES

Fisk, G.R. (1944) The fractured femoral shaft: new approach to the problem. *Lancet*, **i,** 659.
Gunston, F.H. (1971) Polycentric knee arthroplasty. *Journal of Bone and Joint Surgery*, **53–B,** 272.
Strange, F.G. St C. (1965) *The Hip*, p. 99, Fig. iv.6 and p. 269, Fig. x.7. London: Heinemann.
Thomas, H.O. (1876) *Diseases of the Hip, Knee and Ankle Joints, with Their Deformities, Treated by a New and Efficient Method*, 2nd edn, p. 98 and Plate 13, Fig. 4. Liverpool: Dobb.

3.

Fixed traction

If traction is applied to a limb, counter-traction acting in the opposite direction must be applied also, to prevent the body from being pulled in the direction of the traction force. When counter-traction acts through an appliance which obtains a purchase on a part of the body, the arrangement is called fixed traction.

FIXED TRACTION IN A THOMAS'S SPLINT

Fixed traction in a Thomas's splint can 'maintain', but *not* 'obtain' the reduction of a fracture. It is therefore indicated when the femoral fracture can be reduced by manipulation. A reduced transverse fracture is most suitable, but the reduction of an oblique or spiral fracture can be maintained also.

When the cords attached to the adhesive strapping or a tibial Steinmann pin are pulled tight, the counter-thrust passes up the side bars of the splint to the padded ring around the root of the limb (Fig. 3.1). The ring, which must be a snug fit, may cause pressure sores unless daily attention is paid to.the skin (see Ch. 8). The pressure of the padded ring around the root of the limb can be reduced partly by pulling on the end of the splint. A traction weight of 5 lb (2.3 kg) attached to the Thomas's splint usually is sufficient for this purpose.

The significant feature of fixed traction is that the traction force balances the pull of the muscles and, as the muscular pull and haematoma decrease, the traction force decreases. Distraction at the fracture site and the accompanying danger of delayed union or non-union of the fracture is less likely to occur. It is not necessary in this system repeatedly to tighten the traction cords with a windlass, except to compensate for any stretching of the cords or sliding downwards of the adhesive strapping if skin traction is employed.

As counter-traction is not dependant upon gravity the apparatus is self-contained, and the patient may be lifted and moved without risk of displacement of the fracture. This method is valuable in the treatment of civilian casualties. During the Second World War a modification of this method was employed. Skin traction was applied, and while moderate traction was maintained, the

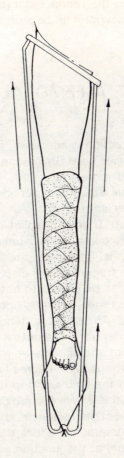

Fig. 3.1   Fixed traction in a Thomas's splint. The grip on the leg is obtained by adhesive strapping.

Note:

— the ring of the Thomas's splint is well up in the groin and fits snugly around the root of the limb.

— the malleoli are well padded to avoid pressure.

— the outer traction cord passes above and the inner cord passes below its respective side bar, to hold the limb in medial rotation.

— the traction cords are tied over the end of the Thomas's splint.

— a windlass is omitted. This avoids the temptation to repeatedly tighten the traction cords and thereby either distract the fracture or pull the adhesive strapping off the limb.

— the counter thrust (traction) passes up the side bars, as indicated by the arrows, to the root of the limb.

lower limb was encased in a skin-tight plaster-of-Paris cast extending from the groin to the toes with the foot at a right angle. Two large holes were cut in the region of the malleoli to allow exit of the skin traction. A Thomas's splint was threaded over the cast and the skin traction tied to the lower end of the splint.

The plaster cast was then split and the splint secured to the cast by bandaging. This assembly was known as the Tobruk splint (Bristow, 1943).

For comfort and ease of movement of the patient, the Thomas's splint can be suspended (see Ch. 5).

REDUCTION OF A FEMORAL SHAFT FRACTURE

For children skin traction is adequate, but for adults skeletal traction with an upper tibial Steinmann pin (Denham pin for the elderly) is used more frequently.

— Insert an upper tibial Steinmann pin under general anaesthesia and attach a Böhler stirrup.

— Thread the prepared Thomas's splint over the limb.

— Palpate the dorsalis pedis and posterior tibial pulses.

— Study the radiographs. Determine the type of fracture, in which direction the fragments are displaced and in which direction they need to be moved to obtain apposition of the bone ends. The next step depends upon the type of fracture.
Transverse fracture. An assistant standing at the foot of the splint holds the Böhler stirrup, exerts a traction force in the long axis of the limb, and simultaneously forces the ring of the splint against the ischial tuberosity.

— Stand at the side of the limb and grip the limb above and below the fracture site. Move the proximal and distal fragments in the directions determined from the study of the pre-reduction radiographs, to reduce the fracture. For example, in a fracture at the junction of the middle and lower thirds of the shaft of the femur, the distal fragment usually is displaced posteriorly. Therefore place one hand under the distal fragment and the other on top of the proximal fragment, and push anteriorly with the hand under the distal fragment. The general rule is that the distal fragment is reduced to the proximal fragment and not vice versa, as the manipulator has control only of the distal fragment, the proximal fragment being under control of the muscles attached to it.

— Check that apposition of the fragments has been obtained by temporarily reducing the traction force. The absence of telescoping of the limb indicates that apposition has been achieved.

— When apposition has been obtained, carefully lower the limb, while maintaining traction, onto the prepared Thomas's splint, with the large pad under the lower part of the thigh.

— Maintain traction.
— Arrange the tension in the other slings to allow 15–20° of knee flexion.
— Attach traction cords to each end of the Steinmann pin and tie them to the lower end of the Thomas's splint.
— Release the pull on the Böhler stirrup.
— Take antero-posterior and lateral radiographs to check the reduction of the fracture. If the reduction is not satisfactory, re-manipulate.
— Palpate the dorsalis pedis and posterior tibial pulses. If the pulses are absent, reduce the traction force. If the pulses do not return, *very gently* re-manipulate the fracture. *If the peripheral pulses are still absent, notify more senior colleagues immediately.*
— If the peripheral pulses are present and the reduction is satisfactory, remove the Böhler stirrup.
— Suspend the Thomas's splint (see Ch. 5).
  Oblique, spiral or comminuted fractures. A formal manipulation of these fractures is not required. The traction force is applied in the long axis of the limb as described above, until the fractured femur is restored to its correct length. Traction is maintained until the traction cords are tied to the foot of the Thomas's splint.
    The instructions about the large pad, radiographs, peripheral pulses and suspension of the Thomas's splint also apply.

TRACTION UNIT

For many years, Charnley (1970), has employed what he terms a traction unit (Fig. 3.2), in conjunction with fixed traction in a Thomas's splint, for the management of fractures of the femoral shaft. Basically a traction unit consists of an upper tibial Steinmann pin incorporated in a light below-knee plaster cast.

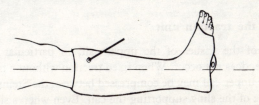

Fig. 3.2   Traction unit. The broken line shows the position of the side bars of the Thomas's splint in relation to the cross-bar fixed to the sole of the plaster cast.

APPLICATION OF A TRACTION UNIT WITH FIXED TRACTION

— Choose the correct size of Thomas's splint.
— Fashion one sling and a large pad to support the thigh.
— Under general anaesthesia, thread the prepared Thomas's splint over the limb, insert an upper tibial Steinmann pin and attach a Böhler stirrup.
— While the leg is supported by an assistant holding the stirrup and keeping the foot at a right angle, apply a padded below-knee plaster cast incorporating the Steinmann pin. The cast must be well padded around the heel to prevent pressure sores from developing.
— Incorporate a 6 inch (15.0 cm) long wooden bar transversely in the sole of the plaster cast about mid-way between the heel and the toes. This bar controls rotation of the limb.
— When the plaster cast has hardened, reduce the fracture and lower the limb on to the prepared splint.
— Check that the thigh sling and the large pad correctly support the thigh, maintaining the normal anterior bowing of the femoral shaft.
— Allow the transverse bar to rest on the side bars of the Thomas's splint. If the thigh sling is correctly tensioned, and the transverse bar is positioned correctly, the knee should be in 15–20° of flexion, and the limb in neutral rotation.
— Attach a cord to each end of the Steinmann pin, loop them once around the side bars of the splint and tie them over the end of the splint.
— Check that the pressure of the thigh sling against the thigh is not excessive. If it is, reduce the pressure by placing a sling under the upper end of the traction unit. The tighter the calf sling is pulled, the more the pressure on the thigh is relieved.
— Suspend the Thomas's splint (Charnley used Method 2, Ch. 5).
— Attach a 5 lb (2.3 kg) weight to the end of the Thomas's splint to reduce partly the pressure of the padded ring of the splint around the root of the limb.

Advantages of the traction unit

1. Compression of the tissues of the upper calf, in particular the common peroneal nerve, does not occur. When fixed traction without a traction unit is employed, the upper calf may be compressed between the Steinmann pin and the upper edge of the sling supporting the calf. Even when a sling is used to support the traction unit, compression of the calf does not occur because it is protected by the plaster cast.

2. Equinus deformity at the ankle cannot occur because the foot is supported by the plaster cast.
3. The tendo calcaneus is protected from pressure by the padded cast.
4. Rotation of the foot and the distal fragment is controlled.
5. A fracture of the ipsilateral tibia can be treated conservatively at the same time as the femoral fracture.

ROGER ANDERSON WELL-LEG TRACTION

Well-leg traction (Anderson, 1932) was originally used in the management of fractures of the pelvis, femur and tibia, skeletal traction being applied to the injured leg, while the 'well' leg was employed for counter-traction. It is rarely used for these purposes today. This method however is valuable in correcting either an abduction or adduction deformity at the hip, for instance before an extra-articular arthrodesis is carried out.

The principle is as follows:

With an abduction deformity at the hip, the affected limb appears to be longer. When traction is applied to the 'well' limb and the affected limb is simultaneously pushed up (counter-traction), the abduction deformity is reduced. Reversing the arrangement will reduce an adduction deformity (Fig. 3.3).

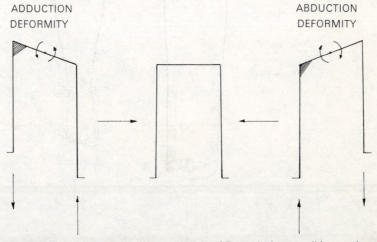

Fig. 3.3   Diagrammatic illustration of the principle of Roger Anderson well-leg traction.

APPLICATION OF ROGER ANDERSON WELL-LEG TRACTION

The simultaneous pulling down of one leg and the pushing up of the other is achieved by using the apparatus illustrated in Figure 3.4.

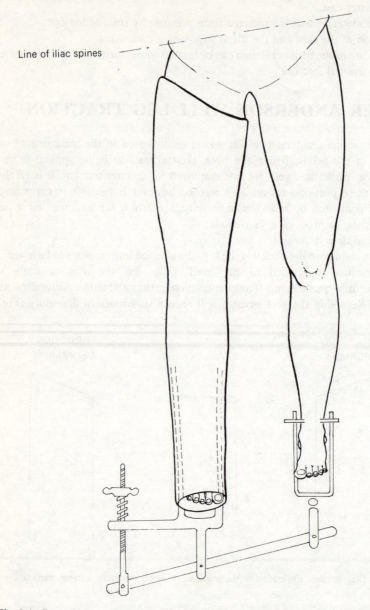

Line of iliac spines

Fig. 3.4 Roger Anderson well-leg traction (modified). The padded below-knee plaster cast is not illustrated.

— Apply an above-knee plaster cast to the limb which is to be pushed upwards. This plaster cast must extend to the top of the thigh; it must be well padded and moulded over the medial aspect of the upper thigh, to prevent the cast pressing on the tissues and obstructing the circulation; and it must be well padded around the ankle and heel as these will be the sites of continuous pressure from the direction of the heel.

— Incorporate the larger stirrup in this plaster.

— Insert a Steinmann pin through the lower end of the tibia of the limb which is to be pulled down, and incorporate the Steinmann pin in a light padded below-knee plaster cast.

— Pass the ends of the Steinmann pin through the lowest possible holes in the side arms of the smaller stirrup.

By altering the position of the screw (on the left in Fig. 3.4), the relative positions of the two stirrups can be altered.

The arrangement illustrated in Figure 3.4 can be used to correct an abduction deformity at the right hip, or an adduction deformity at the left hip.

REFERENCES

Anderson, R. (1932) A new method of treating fractures, utilizing the well leg for counter traction. *Surgery, Gynaecology and Obstetrics,* **54,** 207.

Bristow, W.R. (1943) Some surgical lessons of the war. *Journal of Bone and Joint Surgery,* **25,** 524.

Charnley, J. (1970) *The Closed Treatment of Common Fractures,* 3rd edn, p. 179. Edinburgh: Churchill Livingstone.

4.

Sliding traction

In 1839, John Haddy James of Exeter described a method, which he had employed for several years, of treating fractures of the lower limb with 'continuous yet tolerable traction . . . by weight and pulley' (Jones, 1953). The patient's trunk was fixed to the head of the bed by a rib bandage. The leg was bandaged into a padded hollow splint fitted with a foot piece. A castor on the hollow splint rested upon a wooden plank. A cord from the footpiece passed over a pulley at the foot of the bed to a weight. The head of the bed was raised. James did not utilize the weight of the body, acting under the influence of gravity, to provide counter-traction. In his system, counter-traction was represented by the tension in the rib bandage.

When the weight of all or part of the body, acting under the influence of gravity, is utilized to provide counter-traction, the arrangement is called sliding traction. The traction force is applied by a weight, attached to adhesive strapping or a steel pin by a cord acting over a pulley (Fig. 4.1). The traction force continues to act as long as the weight remains clear of the floor. Counter-traction is obtained by raising one end of the bed by means of wooden blocks or a bed

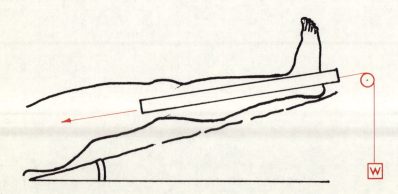

Fig. 4.1 The principle of sliding traction.

elevator, so that the body tends to slide in the opposite direction to that of the traction force.

When sliding traction is used to reduce a fracture, the initial traction weight required to obtain the reduction is greater than the traction weight required to maintain the reduction. *Great care must be taken to ensure that distraction of the fracture does not occur.* For this reason the length of the fractured bone must be measured daily with a tape measure and compared with the normal side, until the correct length has been obtained. When this has been achieved, the traction weight must be reduced to that sufficient to maintain the reduction. Daily radiographic examination may be employed, *but do not ignore the use of a tape measure.*

The traction weight needed to reduce or to maintain the reduction of a particular fracture depends upon the site of the fracture, the age and weight of the patient, the power of his muscles, the amount of muscle damage present and the degree of friction present in the system. The exact weight required is determined by trial, and observing the behaviour of the fracture. For a fracture of the femoral shaft an initial weight of 10% of the weight of the patient is usually sufficient. The heavier the traction weight used, the higher the end of the bed must be raised to provide adequate counter-traction, a rough guide being 1 inch (2.5 cm) for each 1 lb (0.46 kg) of traction weight.

BUCK'S TRACTION OR EXTENSION

Buck's traction, popularised in the American Civil War (Buck, 1861) is used in the temporary management of fractures of the femoral neck; in the management of fractures of the femoral shaft in older and larger children; undisplaced fractures of the acetabulum; after reduction of a dislocation of the hip; to correct minor fixed flexion deformities of the hip or knee; and in place of pelvic traction in the management of low back pain.

APPLICATION OF BUCK'S TRACTION

— Apply adhesive strapping to above the knee or, in elderly patients, with atrophic skin, Ventfoam Skin Traction Bandage.
— Support the leg on a soft pillow to keep the heel clear of the bed.
— Pass the cord from the spreader over a pulley attached to the end of the bed.
— Attach 5 to 7 lb (2.3–3.2 kg) to the cord.
— Elevate the foot of the bed.
    Lateral rotation of the limb is not controlled by this method of traction.

PERKINS TRACTION

Perkins traction can be used in the treatment of fractures of the tibia and of the femur from the subtrochanteric region distally in all age groups, and of trochanteric fractures of the femur in patients aged under 45 to 50 years.

The basis of management of a fracture by Perkins traction is essentially the use of skeletal traction, without any form of external splintage, coupled with active movements of the injured limb which are commenced as soon as possible.

Perkins (1970) considered that traction aligned the fragments, neutralized the pull of the muscles and prevented rotation and angulation at the fracture site, provided that the fracture site was bridged by the origins of a muscle. He believed that by encouraging early muscular activity, the development of stiff joints was frequently prevented by both maintaining extensibility of muscles by reciprocal innervation, and preventing stagnation of tissue fluid; compression at the fracture site occurred which promoted union; and the functional 'severance of the connection between the brain and the damaged limb' was prevented.

Buxton (1981) reported on the results obtained in 50 patients with fractures of the femoral shaft treated by Perkins traction. 47 patients (94%) were in traction for 12 weeks. The remaining three were in traction for a total of 16, 18 and 28 weeks respectively. All 50 patients had at least 120° of knee flexion when traction was discontinued.

A Hadfield split bed*, in which the distal one third of the mattress and the base of the bed can be removed to facilitate flexion of the knee, is required when a fracture of the femur is being treated. Some standard hospital beds can be suitably modified. Fractures of the tibia can be treated in an ordinary standard bed.

A Denham pin is inserted through the upper end of the tibia for fractures of the femur, the mid tibia for fractures of the condyles of the tibia, with the proviso that the pin must be at least one inch (2.5 cm) below the lowest limit of the haematoma resulting from the fracture, and the os calcis for other fractures of the tibia. Denham collars (Fig. 2.6) to which the traction cords are hooked, are attached to the ends of the pins. This method of attaching traction cords to the Denham pins can result in movement being imparted to the pins, causing loosening and infection. New low friction swivels* (Fig. 4.2) have been developed (Simonis, 1980) to overcome this problem.

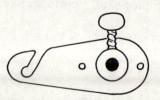

Fig. 4.2 Simonis low friction swivel.

---

*See Appendix.

APPLICATION OF PERKINS TRACTION

1. For fractures of the femur

A Hadfield split bed or a suitably modified standard hospital bed is required.

— Under general anaesthesia and full aseptic conditions, insert a Denham pin through the upper end of the tibia (see pp. 4–10).

— Attach a Simonis swivel to each end of the Denham pin.

— Connect two traction cords, one to each swivel.

— Keeping the traction cords parallel, pass each cord over a separate pulley at the foot of the bed.

— Attach a weight to each traction cord. For the average adult, a 10 lb (4.6 kg) weight is attached to EACH cord making a total traction weight of 20 lb (9.2 kg). This weight is usually reduced to 15 lb (6.9 kg) in the less bulky male patient after about one to two weeks.

— Elevate the foot of the bed by one inch (2.5 cm) for each 1 lb (0.46 kg) of traction weight.

— Place one or more pillows under the thigh to maintain the normal anterior bowing of the femoral shaft. This bowing must, if anything, be accentuated.

— Check the length of the limb with a tape measure, and increase or decrease the total traction weight as necessary.

— Adjust the height of one pulley if necessary to correct rotation.

— Arrange for a radiograph to be taken.

— Start active quadriceps exercises immediately unless precluded from doing so by other injuries and the general condition of the patient.

— Commence knee flexion under supervision of a physiotherapist, about one week after admission, by which time good quadriceps contraction should be present.

— With the injured limb supported, split the bed.

— Place a hand under the patient's heel and encourage him to actively flex his knee as far as possible against resistance. Continue for about 15 minutes on the first day.

— Each day as the patient gains more confidence and more muscular control and requires less manual support, increase the time spent carrying out exercises, reaching a maximum of seven to eight hours per day after two weeks.

2. For fractures of the tibia

Tibial fractures can be nursed in an ordinary standard hospital bed, with the leg resting on a pillow.

— Under general anaesthesia and full aseptic conditions, insert a Denham pin through the selected site (see pp. 4–10).
— Attach a Simonis swivel to each end of the Denham pin.
— Connect two traction cords, one to each swivel.
— Keeping the cords parallel, pass each cord over a separate pulley at the foot of the bed.
— Attach a 5 lb (2.3 kg) weight to EACH cord, making a total traction weight of 10 lb (4.6 kg).
— Elevate the foot of the bed by one inch (2.5 cm) for each 1 lb (0.46 kg) of traction weight.
— Arrange for a radiograph to be taken.
— Start active ankle movements immediately and knee flexion as soon as the patient is able to do so.

HAMILTON RUSSELL TRACTION

Hamilton Russell traction (Russell, 1924) is used in the management of fractures of the femoral shaft and after arthroplasty operations on the hip.

APPLICATION OF HAMILTON RUSSELL TRACTION

See Figure 4.3.
— Apply skin traction to the limb below the knee.
— Attach a pulley to the spreader.

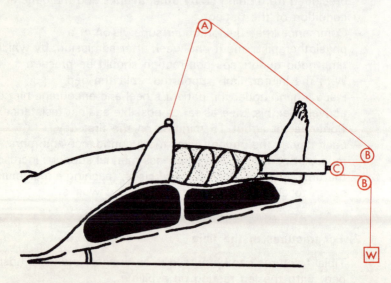

Fig. 4.3 Hamilton Russell traction.

— Place a soft broad sling under the knee.
— Support the limb, with the knee slightly flexed, on two soft pillows, one above and the other below the knee, with the heel clear of the bed.
— Attach a length of cord to the knee-sling.
— Pass the cord over pulley A which is placed well distal to, *not* proximal to the knee, round one of the pulleys B, round pulley C and then around the other pulley B before attaching it to a weight. The pulleys B must be at the same level as the foot of the patient when the leg is lying horizontally on a pillow (Fig. 4.3).
— Elevate the foot of the bed.
Suggested weights:
Adults — 8 lb (3.6 kg).
Infants and older children — $\frac{1}{2}$–4 lb (0.28–1.8 kg).

THEORY OF HAMILTON RUSSELL TRACTION (Fig. 4.4)

The two pulley blocks B at the foot of the bed nominally double the pull on the limb. In practice the pull is modified by the friction present in the system. The resultant of the two forces acting along the cord provides a pull in the line of the shaft of the femur.

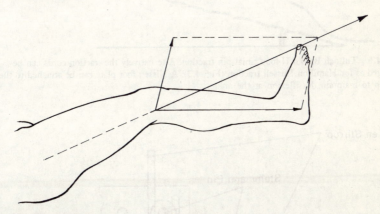

Fig. 4.4 Theory of Hamilton Russell traction. The construction of a parallelogram of forces shows that the resultant force acts in the line of the femoral shaft.

TULLOCH BROWN TRACTION

Tulloch Brown, or U-loop tibial pin, traction and suspension (Nangle, 1951) with a Nissen foot plate and stirrup (Nissen, 1971), is used for the management of patients who have had a cup arthroplasty or pseudarthrosis operation on the hip, or who have sustained a fracture of the shaft of the femur. It is not used in children.

APPLICATION OF TULLOCH BROWN TRACTION

See Figure 4.5.
— Insert a Steinmann pin through the upper end of the tibia.
— Support the leg on slings suspended from the light duralumin U-loop which is slipped over the ends of the Steinmann pin.
  Note: The proximal ends of the U-loop have two staggered lines of holes (Figs 4.5 and 4.7). This arrangement gives a wide choice in the mode of attachment of the U-loop to the

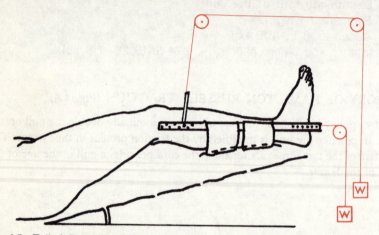

Fig. 4.5 Tulloch Brown U-loop tibial pin traction. Alternatively the traction cords can be arranged as for Hamilton Russell traction (Fig. 4.3). A Nissen foot plate can be attached to the U-loop to maintain dorsiflexion at the ankle.

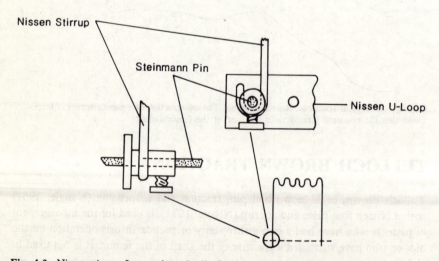

Fig. 4.6 Nissen stirrup. Inserts show detail of attachment to the Steinmann pin.

Steinmann pin. By varying the holes used, it is possible to ensure that the U-loop lies evenly on each side of the leg.

Care must be taken that the slings supporting the calf are not tight, otherwise compression of the tissues of the leg will occur between the proximal edge of the sling nearest the knee, and the Steinmann pin.

— Attach the Nissen stirrup (Fig. 4.6) to the Steinmann pin. This stirrup enables the leg to be suspended and rotation of the limb to be controlled.

— Mount the detachable Perspex foot plate on the U-loop to support the foot (Fig. 4.7). The foot plate prevents equinus of the ankle. In addition, as the attachment of the foot plate to the U-loop is not rigid, the leg muscles can be exercised.

— Use a simple pulley (Fig. 4.5) or Hamilton Russell system (Fig. 4.3) for suspension.

— Elevate the foot of the bed.

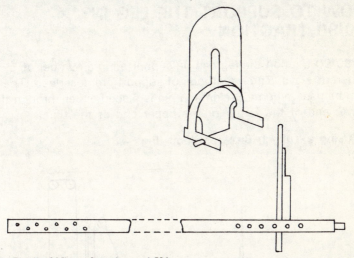

Fig. 4.7 Detail of Nissen foot plate and U-loop.

NINETY/NINETY TRACTION

Ninety/ninety traction was originally devised by Obletz (1946) as an aid to the operative and early post-operative management of compound fractures of the femur with wounds of the posterior aspect of the thigh, sustained in the battles in North Africa during World War II.

Subtrochanteric fractures and those in the proximal third of the shaft of the femur can be difficult to manage in a Thomas's splint because the proximal fragment tends to be flexed and abducted by the muscles attached to it. Although the distal fragment can be aligned with the proximal fragment, the position is frequently lost because of the patient moving in bed. Management of these fractures and compound fractures of the femur with posterior wounds, is easier with 90/90 traction in which the hip and the knee joints are both flexed to 90 degrees.

Skeletal traction is applied either through the lower end of the femur, which is more efficient, or through the upper end of the tibia. It can be used in the management of fractures in children as well as adults. In children, great care must be taken to avoid damage to the epiphyseal growth plates.

Humberger and Eyring (1969) reported on the use of 90/90 traction in the treatment of eighty-one fractures of the shaft of the femur in children, with skeletal traction through the upper end of the tibia. They did not find any evidence of injury to or growth disturbance of the proximal tibial epiphysis, limitation of movement or instability of the knee or cases of ischaemic contracture. They did observe however that children over the age of ten years, or those who weighed in excess of 99 lb (45 kg) tended to develop pain in the knee after about four weeks in traction. They therefore do not recommend the use of 90/90 traction with an upper tibial pin in such children.

HOW TO SUPPORT THE LEG IN 90/90 TRACTION

In 90/90 traction the leg can be supported in a number of different ways. Three methods of support are described. They can be used when a Steinmann pin is placed either through the lower end of the femur or the upper end of the tibia.

1. Using a Tulloch Brown U-loop (Fig. 4.8)

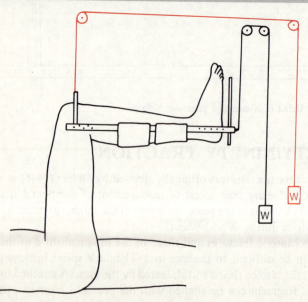

Fig. 4.8 90/90 traction using Tulloch Brown U-loop.

— Fit a Tulloch Brown U-loop (see p. 32) to the Steinmann pin.
— Arrange padded slings to support the calf. Take great care, especially if an upper tibial Steinmann pin is used, that the tissues of the calf are not compressed.
— Attach a Nissen foot plate.
— Tie a cord to the loop at the distal end of the U-loop, and pass it vertically upwards over a pulley.
— Attach sufficient weight to this cord to keep the leg suspended with the knee flexed to 90 degrees.

2. Using a second Steinmann pin (Fig. 4.9)

— Insert a second Steinmann pin through the lower end of the tibia (see p. 9), and attach a Böhler stirrup.
— Tie a cord to the Böhler stirrup and pass it vertically upwards over a pulley.
— Attach sufficient weight to the cord to keep the leg suspended with the knee flexed to 90 degrees.

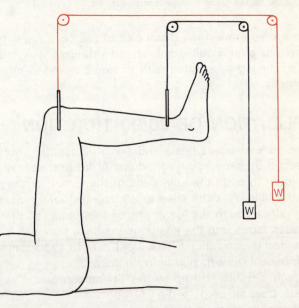

Fig. 4.9 90/90 traction using a second Steinmann through the lower end of the tibia.

3. Using a below-knee plaster cast (Fig. 4.10)

— Apply a below-knee padded plaster cast, incorporating the Steinmann pin, unless a lower femoral pin has been used. The cast must be well padded over the tendo calcaneus and around the malleoli and the back of the heel.

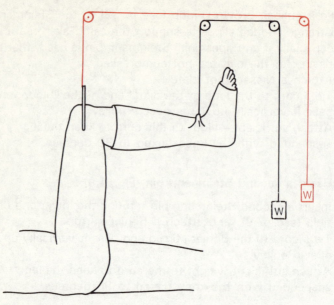

Fig. 4.10 90/90 traction using a below-knee plaster cast.

— Tie a cord around the distal part of the cast, pass it vertically upwards over a pulley and attach sufficient weight to it to keep the leg suspended with the knee flexed to ninety degrees.

APPLICATION OF 90/90 TRACTION

— Use general anaesthesia and take full aseptic precautions.
— Insert a Steinmann pin for adults, or a Kirschner wire for children through the lower end of the femur, or the upper end of the tibia. Flex the knee to 90 degrees before inserting the pin/wire through the lower end of the femur, so that the soft tissues move into the positions in which they will lie when the limb is in traction. Take great care to avoid damage to the epiphyseal growth plates in children.
— Attach a Böhler stirrup to the Steinmann pin.
— Tie a traction cord to the stirrup.
— Choose the method to be used to support the leg (see above).
— Flex the hip and knee joints to ninety degrees.
— Pass the traction cord vertically upwards over a pulley situated above the hip.
— Attach 10–20 lb (4.6–9.2 kg) weight to the traction cord. With unilateral 90/90 traction, the traction weight must not be so great that the buttock on that side is lifted off the bed,

otherwise valgus angulation at the fracture site can occur (Brooker and Schmeisser, 1980).

Varus/valgus angulation at the fracture site is controlled by moving the pulley, over which the traction cord passes, in a plane across the width of the bed.

Rotation is controlled by the knee being flexed, and by ensuring that when the patient is viewed from the foot of the bed, the leg and thigh are in line.

— As union of the fracture occurs, encourage active hip and knee exercises, especially extension, gradually lower the limb into a more horizontal position. As this is done, the foot of the bed may require to be elevated to provide counter-traction.

DANGERS OF NINETY/NINETY TRACTION

1. Those of skeletal traction (see p. 10)
2. Stiffness and loss of extension of the knee
3. Flexion contracture of the hip
4. Injury to the lower femoral or upper tibial epiphyseal growth plates in children
5. Neurovascular damage.

SLIDING TRACTION IN A FISK SPLINT

The treatment of fractures of the femoral shaft and tibial condyles with sliding traction in a Fisk splint (Fig. 2.6) differs from other conservative methods (Fisk, 1944). With fixed traction in a Thomas's splint the knee is held in almost full extension, and little movement is possible. With sliding traction in a Thomas's splint with a knee-flexion piece, some active flexion and extension of the knee is possible, but little movement occurs at the hip, which is in flexion. When a Fisk splint is used, the patient, as soon as possible, begins assisted movement of the lower limb, which is moved as one unit as though the patient were walking. Passive movements are not encouraged (see Ch. 5).

Inhibition of muscular contraction is usually present for the first few days, but within two to three weeks powerful contractions are established. While the limb is exercised, variations in the line of the traction cord relative to the long axis of the femur, and angulation at the fracture site occur, but neither appear to adversely influence the result. Clinical union is present at four to six weeks and sound bony union occurs commonly by twelve weeks at which time a wide range of movement at the knee is present.

APPLICATION OF SLIDING TRACTION WITH A FISK SPLINT

— Adjust the splint to accommodate the limb (see Ch. 2).
— Fashion slings to support the thigh and calf.
— Insert an upper tibial Steinmann pin under general anaesthesia for fractures of the femur. Use skin traction for fractures of the tibial condyles.
— Attach a traction cord to each end of the Steinmann pin (Fig. 5.6) and tie these cords, which must be long enough to clear the foot, to a transverse wooden rod about 6 inches (15.0 cm) long.
— Pass the prepared splint over the limb.
— Manipulate the fracture (see Ch. 3).
— Adjust the position of the thigh pad to maintain the normal anterior bowing of the femoral shaft.
— Tie a single cord to the centre of the wooden rod, pass the cord over a pulley at the foot of the bed and attach a weight. After six weeks the initial traction weight is reduced to 6–8 lb (2.7–3.6 kg).
— Suspend the Fisk splint (see Ch. 5).
— Check that the traction cord is in line with the shaft of the femur when the splint is suspended and the hip is flexed 45 degrees.
— Elevate the foot of the bed.

SLIDING TRACTION WITH A THOMAS'S SPLINT AND A KNEE-FLEXION PIECE

Sliding traction in a Thomas's splint with a knee-flexion piece (Fig. 4.11) is often employed to obtain the reduction of an oblique or spiral fracture of the shaft of

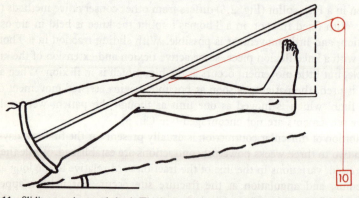

Fig. 4.11 Sliding traction — skeletal. The lower limb rests in a Thomas's splint and a knee-flexion piece. A Steinmann pin is inserted through the upper end of the tibia. A traction cord passes from the pin over a pulley to the traction weight. The foot of the bed is raised to provide counter-traction.

the femur, and then to retain that reduction until union occurs. The use of a knee-flexion piece allows easier mobilisation of the knee. In addition knee flexion controls rotation, prevents stretching of the posterior capsule and posterior cruciate ligament of the knee, which might cause hyperextension instability, and allows variation in the direction of pull when a tibial Steinmann pin is used.

APPLICATION OF SLIDING TRACTION WITH A THOMAS'S SPLINT AND KNEE-FLEXION PIECE

— Choose the correct size of Thomas's splint (see Ch. 2).
— Fashion slings on the knee-flexion piece and the proximal part of the Thomas's splint, and line the slings with Gamgee tissue.
— Insert an upper tibial Steinmann pin.
— Pass the prepared Thomas's splint over the limb, and rest the limb on the padded slings. Remember the large pad under the lower part of the thigh.
— Check that the hinge of the knee-flexion piece lies at the level of the adductor tubercle of the femur.
— Suspend the distal end of the knee-flexion piece by two cords, one on each side, from the distal end of the Thomas's splint. The length of cord is such that the knee is flexed 20–30 degrees. (The extended position is regarded as zero degrees and flexion is measured from this starting position — American Academy of Orthopaedic Surgeons, 1965.) With a supracondylar fracture of the femur, the distal fragment is usually tilted anteriorly upon the shaft. To correct anterior tilting, knee flexion is increased, the amount of knee flexion required being determined radiographically. The end of the knee-flexion piece may be suspended independently by a cord attached to a weight (see Ch. 5). This arrangement allows greater freedom of knee movement.
— Suspend the Thomas's splint (see Ch. 5).
— Adjust the position of the thigh pad and the tension in the sling supporting the pad to obtain the normal anterior bowing of the femoral shaft.
— Attach a Böhler stirrup and cord to the Steinmann pin.
— Pass the cord over a pulley at the foot of the bed so that the cord is in line with the shaft of the femur.
— Attach a weight to the cord.
— Bandage the thigh into the Thomas's splint.
— Elevate the foot of the bed.

SLIDING TRACTION WITH A 'FIXED' THOMAS'S SPLINT

When sliding traction with a Thomas's splint is employed in the treatment of a fracture of the shaft of the femur, there is a tendency for the splint to slip down the limb. This can be avoided by the careful arrangement of the suspension cords (see Ch. 5) or by fixing the traction cords from the patient to the splint, and then pulling on the splint. By this means the traction force passes via the splint to the lower limb (Strange, 1972). A knee-flexion piece is not used.

APPLICATION OF SLIDING TRACTION WITH A 'FIXED' THOMAS'S SPLINT (Strange, 1972)

See Figure 4.12.
— Choose the correct size of Thomas's splint (see Ch. 2).
— Pass the Thomas's splint over the limb while maintaining gentle manual traction.
— Under local or general anaesthesia, insert a Steinmann pin through the upper end of the tibia.
— Attach the traction cords to the Steinmann pin using clamps.
— Twist the cords twice around the side bars of the Thomas's splint.
— Push the Thomas's splint into the groin as far as possible and at the same time apply gentle steady traction to the cords. This achieves the optimal position.
— Tie the cords over the distal end of the Thomas's splint using a reef knot.
— Loop two pieces of tape around each side bar of the Thomas's splint, one at the padded ring, and the other level with the foot.

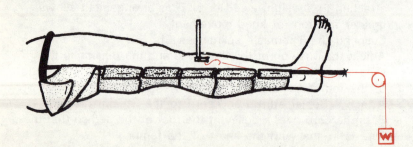

Fig. 4.12   Sliding traction with a 'fixed' Thomas's splint. Note that the Kirschner wire strainer must be kept vertical (Strange, 1972).

— Fashion slings of domette (see Ch. 2) and adjust the tension in the slings to maintain the normal anterior bowing of the shaft of the femur and uniform support of the limb. A thigh pad may be used to maintain the anterior bowing of the shaft of the femur, but its use is not essential.

— Tie a traction cord to the end of the Thomas's splint using a clove hitch, then pass the cord over a pulley at the foot of the bed and attach it to a spring clip.

— Clip a weight to the traction cord. A weight of 18 lb (8.2 kg) is adequate for most adults.

— Suspend the Thomas's splint (see Ch. 5, Method 4) so that the heel is just off the bed, and the traction cord is in line with the splint.

— Elevate the foot of the bed.

BRYANT'S (OR GALLOWS) TRACTION (Fig. 4.13)

Bryant's traction (Bryant, 1880) is convenient and satisfactory for the treatment of fractures of the shaft of the femur in children up to the age of two years who weight less than 35–40 lb (15.9–18.2 kg). Over this age, vascular complications, which are discussed later, may occur.

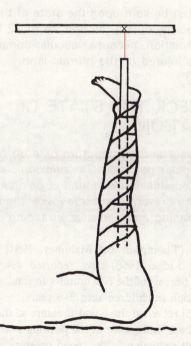

Fig. 4.13 Bryant's (gallows) traction. Note that the child's buttocks are lifted just off the bed. The knees can be kept slightly flexed by applying posterior gutter splints (not illustrated).

APPLICATION OF BRYANT'S TRACTION

— Apply adhesive strapping to *both* lower limbs (shaving is not necessary).
— See below about the use of posterior gutter splints.
— Tie the traction cords to an overhead beam.
— Tighten the traction cords sufficiently to raise the child's buttocks just clear of the mattress. Counter-traction is obtained by the weight of the pelvis and lower trunk.

Children tolerate this position very well, and good alignment of the fracture is obtained. When treating a fracture of the shaft of the femur in a young child, it is preferable to allow the fragments to overlap about ½ inch (1.25 cm), as subsequent overgrowth in length of the femur occurs due to hyperaemia of the limb consequent upon the fracture.

Fractures in children unite rapidly. It is therefore seldom necessary to maintain traction for more than four weeks.

Important: check the state of the circulation in the limbs frequently, because of the danger of vascular complications (see below).

VASCULAR COMPLICATIONS OF BRYANT'S TRACTION

A careful check must be kept upon the state of the circulation in *both limbs,* especially during the first 24 to 72 hours after the application of the traction, because vascular complications may occur in either the injured or the normal limb.

HOW TO CHECK THE STATE OF THE CIRCULATION

— Observe the colour and temperature of *both feet.*
— Dorsiflex *both ankles* passively. *Dorsiflexion should be full and painless.* If dorsiflexion is limited or painful, muscle ischaemia may be present, therefore *lower the limbs and remove all bandaging and adhesive strapping immediately.*

A number of authors (Thompson and Mahoney, 1951; Miller et al, 1952; Nicholson et al, 1955; Lidge, 1959) have reported vascular complications, varying from ischaemic fibrosis of the calf muscles to frank gangrene, following the use of Bryant's traction in children aged 3–8 years.

Nicholson et al, (1955) recorded the blood pressure at the ankles of children aged 1–8 years whose lower limbs were in the position as for Bryant's traction. They found a permanent reduction in the blood pressure at the ankles, which was in almost direct proportion to the hydrostatic pressure necessary to maintain a column of water at the height of the ankles above the heart. This reduction in the blood pressure was particularly proportional in children over the age of two years.

These authors also investigated the influence of hyperextension at the knee on the blood pressure at the ankles. They found, in children under the age of two years, that hyperextension at the knees with or without traction and irrespective of the position of the lower limbs, did not have any appreciable effect upon the blood pressure. In children over the age of 4 years however, the blood pressure at the ankles was reduced to zero when traction was applied with the knees hyperextended and when the lower limbs, without traction but with the knees hyperextended, were raised to the vertical.

Nicholson et al (1955) concluded that in Bryant's traction the blood pressure at the ankles in children under the age of 2 years is insignificantly affected even with hyperextension at the knees; that between the ages of 2 and 4 years the circulation is precarious; and over the age of 4 years the circulation is definitely impaired.

Lidge (1959) stated that the use of Bryant's traction should be limited to children under 4 years old and to those weighing less than 35–40 lb (15.9–18.2 kg).

The use of Bryant's traction is reasonably safe in children under the age of 2 years. Between the ages of 2–4 years vascular complications are more likely to occur, but their occurrence is less likely if posterior gutter splints are applied to keep the knees in slight flexion. Over the age of 4 years the use of Bryant's traction is absolutely contraindicated.

In older children fractures of the shaft of the femur may be adequately treated in Buck's traction or in still older and larger children by fixed traction in a suspended Thomas's splint.

MODIFIED BRYANT'S TRACTION

Modified Bryant's traction (Fig. 4.14) is sometimes used in the initial management of congenital dislocation of the hip when diagnosed over the age of one year. Bryant's traction is set up as described above. After five days abduction of both hips is begun, abduction being increased by about 10 degrees on alternate days. By three weeks the hips should be fully abducted.

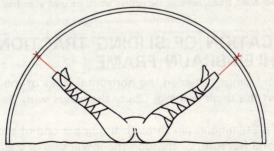

Fig. 4.14 Modified Bryant's traction. The legs initially are vertical. The hips are abducted about 10 degrees on alternate days.

IMPORTANT

1. Check the state of the circulation as described above.

2. Occasionally, after an increase in the degree of abduction of the hips, the child will become restless and scream repeatedly with pain. The pain results from stretching of the capsule of the hip joint by impingement of the femoral head on the superior lip of the acetabulum. This occurs when abduction is commenced before the femoral head has been pulled down to lie opposite the acetabulum. Decreasing the degree of abduction will relieve the pain.

SLIDING TRACTION WITH A BÖHLER-BRAUN FRAME

Sliding traction with a Böhler-Braun frame (Böhler, 1929) can be used for management of fractures of the tibia or femur. It is more commonly used on the continent of Europe. Although skin traction can be employed, skeletal traction is usually used.

The Böhler-Braun frame is illustrated in Figure 4.15. Also indicated are the pulleys over which the cords pass when a femoral or tibial fracture is treated.

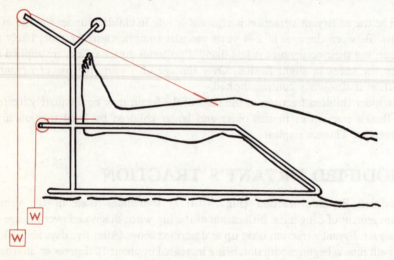

Fig. 4.15 Böhler-Braun frame, showing the pulleys which are used when treating femoral or tibial fractures.

APPLICATION OF SLIDING TRACTION WITH A BÖHLER-BRAUN FRAME

— Suspend slings between the horizontal sides of the frame to support the thigh and leg. Cover the slings with Gamgee tissue.

— Insert a Steinmann pin through the upper end of the tibia for a femoral fracture, or through the lower end of the tibia or the calcaneus for a tibial fracture.

— Attach a Böhler stirrup to the Steinmann pin.
— Place the limb on the slings.
— Attach a cord to the stirrup and pass the cord over the required pulley as shown in Figure 4.15.
— Attach a 7–10 lb (3.2–4.5 kg) weight to the cord.
— Elevate the foot of the bed.

This method of traction has certain disadvantages. The Böhler-Braun frame rests on the patient's bed, and cannot move with the patient. Nursing care is more difficult because the patient is not as mobile as he would be for example in a Thomas's splint. The patient's body and the proximal fragment of the fracture can move relative to the distal fragment which is cradled in the splint and is therefore relatively immobile. This may predispose to the occurrence of a deformity at the fracture site.

LATERAL UPPER FEMORAL TRACTION

Lateral traction through the upper part of the femur can be used either by itself, or in combination with traction in the long axis of the femur (Fig. 4.16), in the management of central fracture-dislocations of the hip, to restore the relationship of the weight-bearing part of the femoral head to the dome of the acetabulum. If only the superior lip of the acetabulum is fractured, Buck's, Hamilton Russell or Tulloch Brown traction is used. If the fracture involves the posterior rim of the acetabulum, and the reduction of the dislocated femoral head is unstable, then vertical skeletal traction through the lower end of the femur or the upper end of the tibia can be used.

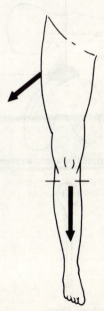

Fig. 4.16 Lateral upper femoral traction combined with traction in the long axis of the femur.

APPLICATION OF LATERAL UPPER FEMORAL TRACTION

— Use general anaesthesia.
— Use full aseptic precautions.
— Do not place a sandbag under either buttock.
— Make a small longitudinal incision centred just below the most prominent part of the greater trochanter.
— Deepen the incision down to bone.
— Identify on the lateral surface of the femur, a point 1 inch (2.5 cm) below the most prominent part of the greater trochanter, and mid-way between the anterior and posterior surfaces of the femur (Fig. 1.8).
— Ask an assistant to rotate the lower limb medially until the patella points vertically upwards. This ensures that the normal forward angulation (anteversion) of the femoral neck is eliminated, and that the femoral neck is lying horizontally (Fig. 4.17).
— Drill a small hole in the lateral cortex of the femur, using the correct size of drill for the coarse-threaded screw, or screw eye (Fig. 4.18) (Zimmer pelvic traction screw*; Zimmer, USA).

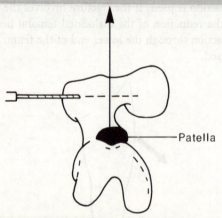

Patella

Fig. 4.17 With the patella pointing vertically upwards, anteversion of the femoral neck is eliminated.

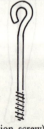

Fig. 4.18 Screw eye (Zimmer pelvic traction screw).

*See Appendix.

- Place a finger over the femoral artery at the groin as this indicates the position of the head of the femur.
- Hold the drill horizontally and direct it cranially towards the finger over the femoral artery.
- Advance the drill $1\frac{1}{2}$–2 inches (3.75–5.0 cm) up the femoral neck.
- Remove the drill.
- Insert the coarse-threaded screw or screw eye.
- Suture the wound.
- Attach a traction cord to the screw eye. If a coarse-threaded screw is used, attach a length of stainless steel wire to the screw and then the traction cord to the stainless steel wire (Fig. 4.19).

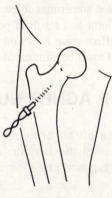

Fig. 4.19 Stainless steel wire attached to a coarse-threaded screw to obtain lateral upper femoral traction.

- Pass the traction cord over a pulley at the side of the bed.
- Attach 10–20 lb (4.5–9.0 kg) to the traction cord.
- Tilt the patient's bed, raising it on the affected side to produce counter-traction. If lateral upper femoral traction is used in combination with traction in the long axis of the femur, the patient's bed will require to be tilted in two planes, the foot of the bed being highest on the affected side and the head of the bed lowest on the unaffected side (Fig. 4.20).
- Encourage active movements of the hip and knee. Lateral traction through the upper end of the femur is continued for 4–6 weeks.

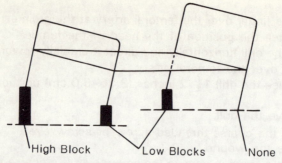

Fig. 4.20 Method of obtaining tilt of the bed in two planes when lateral upper femoral traction is combined with traction in the long axis of the femur.

AGNES HUNT TRACTION FOR THE CORRECTION OF A FLEXION DEFORMITY OF THE HIP

This traction technique is used sometimes to correct a mild flexion deformity that has occurred at the hip joint as a result of poliomyelitis.

For traction to have any effect upon a flexion deformity at a hip joint, the compensatory lumbar lordosis must be eliminated (Duthie and Ferguson, 1973).

APPLICATION OF AGNES HUNT TRACTION
(Fig. 4.21)

— Lie the patient supine on an orthopaedic table.
— Flex both hip joints until the lumbar lordosis is abolished.
— Keep the unaffected hip and knee joints both flexed to ninety degrees.
— Apply a plaster hip spica cast to include the lumbar spine and the unaffected lower limb, but NOT the affected lower limb.

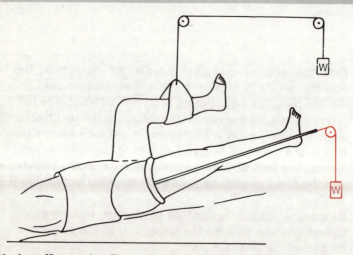

Fig. 4.21 Agnes Hunt traction. The unaffected lower limb is encased in a single hip spica. Skin traction is applied to the affected lower limb which rests in a Thomas's splint.

— Support the encased lower limb with slings and weights.
— Apply skin traction to the affected lower limb.
— Thread a prepared Thomas's splint (see p.14) over the affected lower limb.
— Apply traction with the affected hip initially in flexion. As the flexion deformity decreases, gradually lower the Thomas's splint.
— When the flexion deformity has been corrected, remove the traction, Thomas's splint and hip spica cast.

PELVIC TRACTION

In pelvic traction a special canvas harness is buckled around the patient's pelvis. Long cords or straps attach the harness to the foot of the bed. When the foot of the bed is raised, gravity causes the patient to slide towards the head of the bed. The amount by which the foot of the bed must be elevated depends upon the patient's weight: the heavier the patient, the more the foot of the bed must be raised.

This type of traction is used often in the conservative management of a prolapsed lumbar intervertebral disc. The function of the traction is to ensure that the patient lies quietly in bed, rather than to attempt to distract the vertebral bodies. The vertebral bodies can be distracted by traction, but the pull required is very much greater than that which can be exerted by this arrangement.

Buck's traction, applied to both lower limbs, with the cords attached either to the foot of the bed, or to traction weights, may be employed also in the conservative management of a prolapsed lumbar intervertebral disc. Pelvic traction is superior, however, because it leaves the patient's legs unencumbered and therefore able to move freely.

DUNLOP TRACTION (Fig. 4.22)

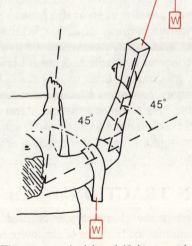

Fig. 4.22 Dunlop traction. The upper arm is abducted 45 degrees, and the elbow is flexed 45 degrees.

Dunlop traction (Dunlop, 1939) is used in the management of supracondylar and transcondylar fractures of the humerus in children. This method is useful especially if flexion of the elbow causes circulatory embarrassment with loss of the radial pulse. Prietto (1979) states that Dunlop traction, in which the forearm is in supination, is best used in the treatment of supracondylar fractures of the humerus where the distal fragment is displaced postero-laterally.

APPLICATION OF DUNLOP TRACTION

— Apply skin traction to the forearm.
— Place the patient supine on the bed.
— Abduct the shoulder about 45 degrees.
— Pass the traction cord over a pulley so placed that the elbow is flexed about 45 degrees.
— Place a padded sling over the distal humerus.
— Attach weights to the traction cord and padded sling, so that the upper arm is just clear of the bed with the elbow in about 45 degrees of flexion. The weights required will depend upon the size of the child but often 1–2 lb (0.5–1.0 kg) is sufficient initially.
— Elevate the same side of the bed as the affected limb and/or pad the side of the cot.
— Under radiographic control, increase the traction weight daily until a satisfactory reduction of the fracture is obtained.
— Check the state of the circulation in the limb at HOURLY intervals for the first twelve hours, and then twice daily while the traction weights are being increased.

Note: It is not sufficient to determine whether the radial pulse is present or not. Check that the child has full active or passive extension of the fingers without pain, and that sensation in the fingers is normal. Ischaemia of the forearm muscles can be present even in the presence of a radial pulse. If ischaemia is present, active extension of the fingers will be absent and passive extension of the fingers will be painful. If ischaemia is suspected, discontinue traction immediately. It is much better to run the risk of mal-union of the fracture than Volkmann's ischaemic contracture of the forearm. If this fails to relieve the circulatory embarrassment, carry out a closed manipulation of the fracture, before proceeding to exploration of the brachial artery or fasciotomy of the forearm.

OLECRANON TRACTION (Figs 4.23, 4.24)

Skeletal traction through the olecranon can be used in the management of supracondylar and comminuted fractures of the lower end of the humerus, and unstable fractures of the shaft of the humerus.

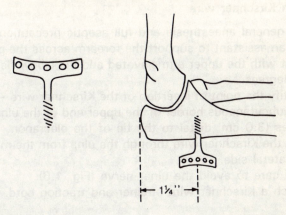

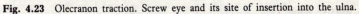

Fig. 4.23 Olecranon traction. Screw eye and its site of insertion into the ulna.

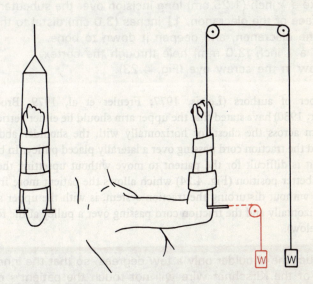

Fig. 4.24 Olecranon traction.

The traction force may be applied either through a Kirschner wire and strainer, or a screw eye* (Ormandy, 1974). The advantages of olecranon traction are that with skeletal traction, a greater force can be applied; rotation at the fracture site can be controlled by moving the forearm around the longitudinal axis of the humerus; and angulation can be corrected by varying the direction of pull of the traction weights.

*See Appendix.

APPLICATION OF OLECRANON TRACTION

1. With Kirschner wire

— Use general anaesthesia and full aseptic precautions.
— Ask an assistant to support the forearm across the patient's chest with the upper arm elevated and the elbow flexed to 90 degrees.
— Identify the point of insertion of the Kirschner wire — deep to the subcutaneous border of the upper end of the ulna, $1\frac{1}{4}$ inches (3.0 cm) distal to the tip of the olecranon.
— Pass the Kirschner wire through the ulna from the medial to the lateral side.
— Take care to avoid the ulnar nerve (Fig. 1.6).
— Attach a Kirschner wire strainer and traction cord.

2. With screw eye

— Use general anaesthesia and full aseptic precautions.
— Make a $\frac{1}{2}$ inch (1.25 cm) long incision over the subcutaneous surface of the olecranon, $1\frac{1}{4}$ inches (3.0 cm) distal to the tip of the olecranon, and deepen it down to bone.
— Drill a $\frac{1}{8}$ inch (3.0 mm) hole through the cortex.
— Screw in the screw eye (Fig. 4.23).

A number of authors (Lewis, 1977; Freuler et al, 1979; Brooker and Schmeisser, 1980) have stated that the upper arm should lie either vertically with the forearm across the chest, or horizontally with the shoulder abducted 45 degrees and the traction cord passing over a laterally placed pulley. In both these positions, it is difficult for the patient to move without upsetting the traction system. A better position (Fig. 4.24) which allows the patient more freedom of movement without disturbing the traction system, is with the upper arm lying almost horizontally and the traction cord passing over a pulley at the foot of the bed (see below).

— Abduct the shoulder only a few degrees, so that the inner end of the Kirschner wire will not touch the patient's chest.
— With the upper arm lying almost horizontally, pass the traction cord over a pulley situated at the foot of the bed.
— Attach the traction weight to the cord — 3–4 lb (1.3–1.8 kg).
— Attach two cords, one to each end of the Kirschner wire, and pass them vertically upwards over two pulleys situated above the elbow.
— Attach 1 to 2 lb (0.5–1.0 kg) to these cords.
— Make a soft loop between these two cords in the region of the wrist, to support the forearm.

- Adjust the weights until the correct alignment is obtained.
- Instruct the patient to fully exercise his fingers and wrist at hourly intervals.
- Check the circulation, sensation and movement of the fingers daily.

Rotation at the fracture site is controlled by moving the pulleys over which the cords from each end of the Kirschner wire pass, either towards or away from the patient. Moving the pulleys towards the patient will cause medial rotation at the fracture site, whereas moving the pulleys away from the patient, will cause lateral rotation.

If a screw eye is used in place of a Kirschner wire and strainer skin traction will have to be applied to the forearm, to support it.

METACARPAL PIN TRACTION

Skeletal traction through the second and third metacarpal bones can be used in the management of comminuted fractures of the bones of the forearm — in particular a comminuted fracture of the lower end of the radius — and in combination with olecranon pin traction for fractures of the humerus and the bones of the forearm in the same limb.

APPLICATION OF METACARPAL PIN TRACTION
(Figs 4.25, 4.26)

- Use general anaesthesia.
- Use full aseptic precautions.
- Ask an assistant to hold the limb by the fingers and forearm.
- Squeeze the hand to increase the transverse metacarpal arch. The fourth and fifth metacarpals are relatively more mobile than the second and third, and therefore increasing the transverse metacarpal arch will move the heads of the fourth and fifth metacarpals towards the palm thus exposing the distal ends of the second and third metacarpals (Fig. 4.25).

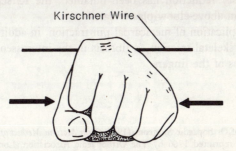

Kirschner Wire

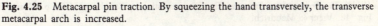

Fig. 4.25 Metacarpal pin traction. By squeezing the hand transversely, the transverse metacarpal arch is increased.

— Insert a Kirschner wire from the radial to the ulnar side,
  through the distal part of the shafts of the second and third
  metacarpals so that the wire is at right angles to the long
  axis of the radius (Fig. 1.7).
— Avoid the metacarpo-phalangeal joints.
— Fit the Kirschner wire strainer, and attach a traction cord.
— Pass the traction cord vertically upwards over a pulley.
— Attach 3–4 lb (1.3–1.8 kg) to the cord.
— Arrange a sling over the upper arm to which the weight can
  be attached to provide counter traction (Fig. 4.26).

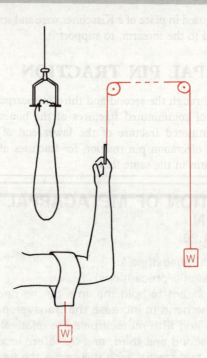

Fig. 4.26   Metacarpal pin traction, using a Kirschner wire strainer, and a canvas sling over the
upper arm to provide counter-traction.

After a satisfactory reduction has been obtained, the Kirschner wire can be
incorporated in an above-elbow plaster cast.

The main complication of metacarpal pin traction, in addition to the general
complications of skeletal traction, is fibrosis in the interosseous muscles which
can cause stiffness of the fingers.

REFERENCES

American Academy of Orthopaedic Surgeons (1965) *Joint Motion: Method of Measuring and
  Recording*, p. 66, reprinted 1966 by The Orthopaedic Association. London: Churchill.
Böhler, L. (1929) *The Treatment of Fractures*. English translation by Steinberg, M.E., p. 34 and
  p. 35, Fig. 48. Vienna: Maudrich.

Brooker, A.F. & Schmeisser, G. (1980) *Orthopaedic Traction Manual.* Baltimore: Williams & Wilkins.

Bryant, T. (1880) On the value of parallelism of the lower extremities in the treatment of hip disease and hip injuries, with the best means of obtaining it. *Lancet,* **i,** 159.

Buck, G. (1861) An improved method of treating fractures of the thigh illustrated by cases and a drawing. *Transactions of the New York Academy of Medicine,* **2,** 232.

Buxton, R.A. (1981) The use of Perkins' traction in the treatment of femoral shaft fractures. *Journal of Bone and Joint Surgery,* **63-B,** 362.

Dunlop, J. (1939) Transcondylar fractures of the humerus in childhood. *Journal of Bone and Joint Surgery,* **21,** 59.

Duthie, R.B. & Ferguson, A.B. (1973) *Mercer's Orthopaedic Surgery,* p. 385. London: Edward Arnold.

Fisk, G.R. (1944) The fractured femoral shaft: new approach to the problem. *Lancet,* **i,** 659.

Freuler, F., Wiedmer, U. & Bianchini, D. (1979) *Cast Manual for Adults and Children.* Berlin: Springer-Verlag.

Humberger, F.W. & Eyring, E.J. (1969) Proximal tibial 90/90 traction in treatment of children with femoral shaft fractures. *Journal of Bone and Joint Surgery,* **51-A,** 499.

Jones, A.R. (1953) John Haddy James. *Journal of Bone and Joint Surgery,* **35-B,** 661.

Lewis, R.C. (1977) *Handbook of Traction, Casting and Splinting Techniques.* Philadelphia: Lippincott.

Lidge, R.T. (1959) Complications following Bryant's traction, in American Medical Association, section on Orthopaedic Surgery, Annual Meeting 1959. *Journal of Bone and Joint Surgery,* **41-A,** 1540.

Miller, D.S., Markin, L. & Grossman, E. (1952) Ischaemic fibrosis in lower extremity in children. *American Journal of Surgery,* **84,** 317.

Nangle, E.J. (1951) *Instruments and Apparatus in Orthopaedic Surgery,* p. 9. Oxford: Blackwell.

Nicholson, J.T., Foster, R.M. & Heath, R.D. (1955) Bryant's traction, a provocative cause of circulatory complications. *Journal of the American Medical Association,* **157,** 415.

Nissen, K.I. (1950) Osteomyelitis of the acetabulum with intrapelvic protrusion of the head of the femur. *Proceedings of the Royal Society of Medicine,* **43,** 306.

Obletz, B.E. (1946) Vertical traction in the early management of certain compound fractures of the femur. *Journal of Bone and Joint Surgery,* **24,** 113.

Ormandy, L. (1974) Olecranon screw for skeletal traction of the humerus. *American Journal of Surgery,* **127,** 615.

Perkins, G. (1970) *The Ruminations of an Orthopaedic Surgeon.* London: Butterworth.

Prietto, C.A. (1979) Supracondylar fractures of the humerus. A comparative study of Dunlop's traction versus percutaneous pinning. *Journal of Bone and Joint Surgery,* **61-A,** 425.

Russell, R.H. (1924) Fractures of the femur: a clinical study. *British Journal of Surgery,* **II,** 491.

Simonis, R.B. (1980) Personal communication.

Strange, F.G.St C. (1972) Personal communication.

Thomson, S.A. & Mahoney, L.J. (1951) Volkmann's ischaemic contracture and its relationship to fractures of the femur. *Journal of Bone and Joint Surgery,* **33-B,** 336.

5.

Suspension of appliances

One initial difficulty in understanding traction is the presence of the many cords attached to both the patient and the appliance. The problem is simplified if it is recognised that the cords perform two distinct and separate functions: traction, described in Chapters 1, 3 and 4, and suspension of the appliance. (In the illustrations, *black* is used for suspension cords, and *red* for traction cords.)

By suspending appliances the mobility of the patient is increased, nursing is easier and the dangers of immobility — thrombosis and embolism, pressure sores, muscle wasting, joint stiffness and contractures, pneumonia, decalcification, renal stones and urinary infection — are decreased.

The appliance is suspended from an overhead frame by a series of counter-weights attached to it by cords which run over pulleys. A Thomas's splint can also be suspended by springs. The overhead frame is generally referred to as a Balkan beam, although each manufacturer uses a different name for his own overhead frame.

THE BALKAN BEAM

Overhead wooden beams were introduced during the Balkan Wars by a Dutch ambulance unit in 1903 (Bick, 1948). Today the Balkan beam is made from metal tubing which may be of round, square or octagonal cross section, depending upon the manufacturer. The methods of fixing the tubing to the bed differ, but the basic principle is the same.

Two uprights, one attached to each end of the bed, are joined by a longitudinal horizontal bar. Other shorter transverse horizontal bars may be attached to the uprights and to the longitudinal horizontal bar.

When a single Thomas's splint is to be suspended, only a single Balkan beam is required. One upright is attached to the centre of the top of the bed, and the other upright is attached to the same side of the foot of the bed as that on which the injured limb lies. If two splints or a plaster bed are to be suspended, two Balkan beams are required. The Balkan beams are attached to each side of the ends of the bed, and are joined together by the transverse horizontal bars.

SUSPENSION CORDS

Sash cord generally is used to suspend appliances. Easier recognition of the function of each cord in a traction-suspension system is possible if cords of two different colours are used, for example, red or green for traction cords, and white for suspension cords.

The cords must be attached firmly to the appliance. If they slip, the efficiency of the system is reduced and the patient may be injured. Many of the remarks made below apply also to the attachment of traction cords.

KNOTS

Clove hitch (Fig. 5.1).
A clove hitch is the best knot to use to attach a cord to an appliance, as it is self tightening and therefore is less likely to slip. It can be reinforced if necessary with a half hitch.

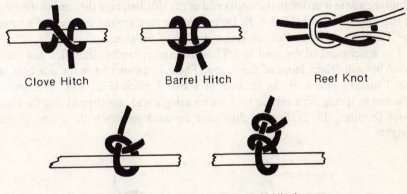

Clove Hitch   Barrel Hitch   Reef Knot

Half Hitch   Two Half Hitches

Fig. 5.1 Clove hitch, barrel hitch, reef knot, half hitch, two half hitches.

Barrel hitch (Fig. 5.1).
A barrel hitch is used to attach a single cord to a loop of cord. The position of the knot on the cord can be altered easily, by sliding the knot along the loop. When the correct position is obtained, the barrel hitch is converted to a reef knot as shown in Figure 5.3.

Reef knot (Fig. 5.1).
The cords used in traction-suspension systems should not be joined, as the knots may jam in the pulleys. If it should be necessary to join two lengths of cord, a reef knot is used.

Half hitch (Fig. 5.1)

Two half hitches (Fig. 5.1)
After a knot is tied, the cord is cut about 2 inches (5.0 cm) away from the knot.

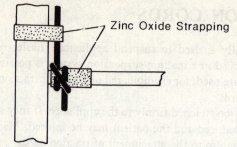

Fig. 5.2 The suspension cord can be taped to the ring of a Thomas's splint to prevent it slipping down the side bar.

The free end can be bound to the main cord with a short length of zinc oxide or similar strapping. The knot itself must not be obscured by the strapping. This further reinforces the attachment of the cord to the appliance.

Even a clove hitch may slip on the side bars of a Thomas's splint. This can be prevented by wrapping a short length of zinc oxide strapping around the side bars over which the knot is tied. To further prevent the suspension cord from slipping, where it is tied to the upper end of the side bar, tape the cord to the ring of the Thomas's splint (Fig. 5.2). Do not tie the cord around the padded ring of the Thomas's splint as this can cause chafing of the skin.

The attachment of the cord to a Thomas's splint can be simplified and time saved by using short loops of linen tape. These loops are tied to the side bars of the Thomas's splint in the manner of a barrel hitch (Fig. 5.1). The cords, attached to spring clips similar to those on a dog's lead, are clipped into the tape loops (Strange, 1972). Spring clips may be used to attach the cords to the weights.

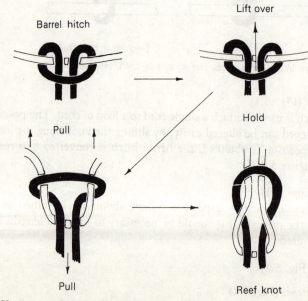

Fig. 5.3 How to convert a barrel hitch into a reef knot.

PULLEYS

The function of a pulley is to control the direction of action of the weight attached to the end of the cord passing over the pulley. By altering the site of attachment of the cord and the pulley, or by using more than one pulley in the system, the force exerted by a given weight can be increased. This is termed the mechanical advantage of the system.

Large pulley wheels of 2–2½ inches (5.0–6.25 cm) diameter and with ¼ inch (6 mm) diameter axles are preferable. Small rough cast pulley wheels, such as used for clothes lines, are less efficient. The majority of pulley wheels supplied by the manufacturers of orthopaedic supplies are made from Tufnol, nylon or a similar synthetic material. All pulleys must be kept clean and oiled where necessary.

A compound pulley block (Fig. 5.4) consists of four small wheels on a common axle and one large wheel on its own axle, all enclosed in a common frame. The frame can be opened at one side to allow the cords to be slipped on and off the wheels. The cords attached to the appliance usually are looped over the smaller wheels, but if a pulley system with an increased mechanical advantage is required, the compound pulley block can be inverted. This arrangement is used in suspending a plaster bed (see p. 68).

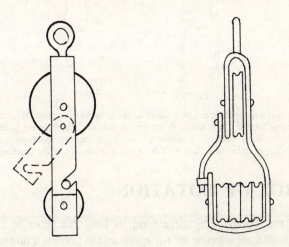

Fig. 5.4 A compound pulley block, used in suspension of a Thomas's splint (Fig. 5.9) and a plaster bed (Fig. 5.12).

When suspending a Thomas's splint, the pulleys must be positioned correctly as the directions in which the cords run from the splint to the pulleys are important. The cords by their direction of pull keep the ring of the splint around the root of the limb, raise the splint off the mattress and thus enable the patient to move freely, and at the same time maintain the splint and thus the distal fragment of the fracture in correct alignment with the proximal fragment (Fig. 5.5).

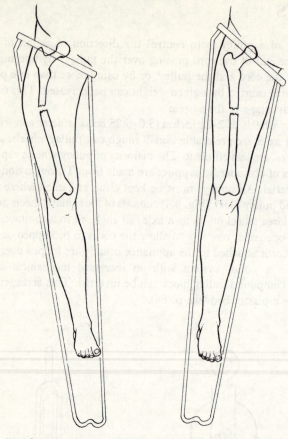

Fig. 5.5 The distal fragment must be reduced to the proximal fragment. With a fracture at the junction of the middle and upper thirds of the femur, the proximal fragment is abducted as well as flexed, while the distal fragment is adducted. The splint, carrying the distal fragment, must therefore be abducted, otherwise there will be a varus deformity at the fracture site.

CONTROL OF ROTATION

Rotation of the Thomas's splint around its long axis must be controlled, to prevent the limb from slipping off the splint and to prevent union of the fracture occurring in mal-rotation. Rotation is most likely to occur in a lateral direction.

The methods employed to control rotation are described below with each individual method of suspension of the Thomas's splint.

SUSPENSION WEIGHTS

The amount of weight required to suspend an appliance depends upon the weight of the appliance, the weight of the part of the body suspended in the appliance, the mechanical advantage of the system employed for suspension, and the amount of friction present in the system.

The actual amount of weight required is determined by observing the behaviour of the suspension system. When the correct amount of weight is obtained, the appliance will move readily in all directions with little effort on the part of the patient, will return quickly to the position of rest, and will maintain the appliance in its correct relationship to the patient.

PREVENTION OF EQUINUS DEFORMITY AT THE ANKLE

When a lower limb is immobilised in recumbency for any length of time, weakness of the muscles of dorsiflexion of the ankle may occur with subsequent contraction of the posterior capsule of the ankle joint and the development of fixed equinus deformity at the ankle.

To reduce the risk of this occurring, active dorsiflexion of the ankle must be commenced immediately and be carried out regularly. The risk can be reduced further by providing a support for the foot. This can be achieved in several ways.

Foot piece
A U-shaped length of metal is clamped to the side bars of the Thomas's splint level with the sole of the foot. The foot rests upon a sling which passes between the limbs of the U-loop.

Stockinette
A length of stockinette, knotted at one end, is pulled over the foot like a sock. A cord, tied to the knotted end of the stockinette is passed cranially over a pulley to a small weight.

Traction unit
In a traction unit the foot is supported by the plaster cast.

Nissen foot plate
In U-loop tibial pin traction and suspension.

Elastic
When a Fisk splint is used, a long length of elastic can be tied to the eyelets of the squared-off frame and passed round the sole of a slipper to which it is stitched.

SUSPENSION OF TULLOCH BROWN TIBIAL U-LOOP

The Tulloch Brown tibial U-loop can be suspended either by using the same arrangement of cord, pulleys and one weight as employed in Russell traction (Fig. 4.3), or by using a simple pulley system and two weights as illustrated in Figure 4.5.

Rotation is controlled by varying the site of attachment of the cord to the Nissen stirrup.

SUSPENSION OF THE FISK SPLINT (Fisk, 1944)

The Fisk splint (see Chs 2, 4) is suspended from three points on an overhead beam. The end of the knee-flexion piece is suspended by a single cord looped over the overhead beam. The length of this cord is such that when the hip is flexed to an angle of 45 degrees, the leg is horizontal. The ends of a second long loop of cord are attached to the eyelets at the corners of the squared-off frame. This second loop passes upwards and cranially over a pulley on the overhead beam, situated over the patient's abdomen. It is attached to a *single* suspension weight of usually 4–8 lb (1.8–3.6 kg) which is passed through the loop by a slip knot, and which hangs within easy reach of the patient. This suspension cord is at right angles to the long axis of the femur when the hip is flexed to an angle of 45 degrees (Fig. 5.6).

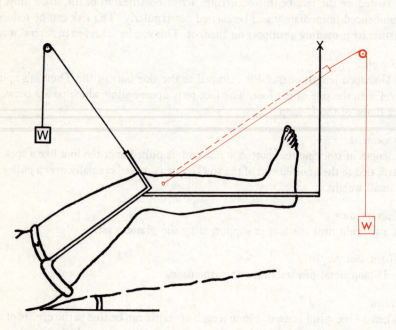

Fig. 5.6 Suspension of the Fisk splint.

The patient flexes his hip, assisting the movement by pulling down on the suspension weight, and at the same time flexes his knee and dorsiflexes his ankle. The patient then actively extends his hip and knee and plantar-flexes his ankle while gradually releasing his pull on the suspension weight. Passive movements are not encouraged.

Rotation is controlled by varying the length of each attachment of the fixed cord to the end of the knee-flexion piece, and by varying the tension in the loop of cord attached to the squared-off frame.

METHODS OF SUSPENDING A THOMAS'S SPLINT

Fracture boards are placed under the mattress to ensure a firm base.

A suspended Thomas's splint is entirely free from the bed, except at its upper end where the back of the padded ring rests on the mattress. The patient can raise his pelvis off the bed by pulling up with his arms on a patient's helper, aided by downward pressure on the bed with his other foot. The whole of the injured limb, from the ischial tuberosity to the foot, moves in one piece with the patient's trunk, and therefore the position of the fracture is unchanged.

USING CORDS, PULLEYS AND WEIGHTS

A Thomas's splint may be suspended in a number of different ways using cords, pulleys and weights. The details differ but the principles are the same.

1. The cords must be attached firmly to the splint. Different methods of attaching the cords to the splint have been described above.

2. The Thomas's splint must not move independently of the lower limb. In fixed traction the counter-traction force is directed up the side bars of the splint (Fig. 3.1), and therefore the ring of the splint remains around the root of the limb. In sliding traction, counter-traction is obtained by raising the foot of the bed to utilize body weight. The splint only supports the limb. If a cranially-directed force is not applied to the splint, the splint may be pulled down the limb with serious consequences for the position of the fracture.

3. The pulleys must be positioned correctly and run smoothly.

4. Rotation of the Thomas's splint must be controlled.

5. The suspension weights must be adjusted carefully.

Method one (Fig. 5.7)
Small loops of cord are formed between the side bars of the splint at each end.

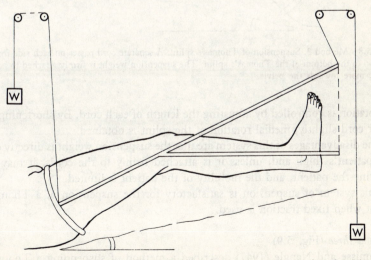

Fig. 5.7   Method 1. Suspension of Thomas's splint. Separate suspension cords and weights are attached to each end of the Thomas's splint.

The suspension cords are attached to the centre of each loop using a barrel hitch, and are then passed upwards and cranially to pulleys. From these pulleys the cords pass to other pulleys situated at the head or foot of the bed, before running vertically down to weights.

Rotation of the splint is adjusted by moving the position of the knots on the proximal and distal loops, until the correct position is obtained, when the barrel hitches are converted to reef knots.

The disadvantages of this system are that the proximal cord passes close to the patient's face, the ring of the splint is not adequately retained in the groin, and the patient's mobility is limited.

Method two (Fig. 5.8)
Two lengths of cord, one on each side, are attached to each end of the splint. Each cord passes over two pulleys. A suspension weight is attached firmly to both cords at a point nearer the pelvis.

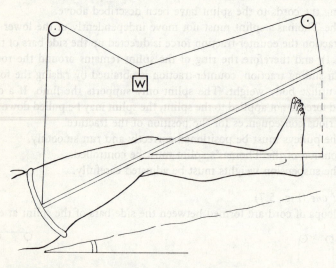

Fig. 5.8 Method 2. Suspension of Thomas's splint. A separate cord passes on each side from the top to the bottom of the Thomas's splint. The suspension weight is firmly attached to both cords, more towards the pelvis.

Rotation is controlled by adjusting the length of each cord. By shortening the outer cord slightly, medial rotation of the splint is obtained.

The disadvantages of this system are that the suspension weight is directly over the patient's thigh and, unless it is attached firmly to the cords, it may fall injuring the patient, and the mobility of the patient is limited.

This system of suspension is satisfactory for the suspension of a Thomas's splint when fixed traction is used.

Method three (Fig. 5.9)
Dommisse and Nangle (1947) described a method of suspending a Thomas's splint using a compound pulley block.

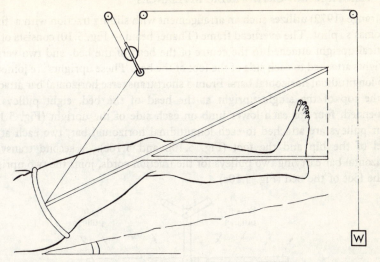

Fig. 5.9 Method 3. Suspension of a Thomas's splint. A compound pulley block (Fig. 5.4) is used. Two cords pass from top to bottom of the splint, one on each side, passing over the smaller wheels of the compound pulley block.

Two lengths of cord, one on each side, are attached to each end of the splint. These cords must not be too long. Both cords pass over the smaller wheels of a compound pulley block, situated over the patient's thigh. A cord passes up from the ring above the larger wheel, over a pulley attached to the overhead frame, down and round the larger wheel of the compound pulley block and then up again and round a second pulley before passing towards the foot of the bed. There the cord passes over another pulley before running vertically down to a weight. The arrangement of the pulleys and cords produces a suspension system with a mechanical advantage of three to one. A suspension weight of 8 lb (3.6 kg) is usually adequate.

In this arrangement the splint pivots around the smaller wheels of the compound pulley block, the height of which can vary. If the proximal end of the splint is raised and the distal end lowered, the pulley block moves proximally, and the force directed cranially is increased, thus preventing the splint from slipping down the leg.

If the front of the ring of the splint presses upon the patient's thigh, the pulleys attached to the overhead frame are moved cranially.

Rotation of the splint is controlled by varying the length of the cords attached to each end of the splint. Further fine adjustment is obtained by varying the position of the cords on the smaller wheels of the pulley block.

This is an excellent system of suspension and it can be used with either fixed or sliding traction.

Method four
Setting up the suspension systems described above takes time. The time taken can be reduced considerably if a bed with an overhead frame, pulleys, cords and weights is prepared beforehand.

Strange (1972) utilizes such an arrangement with sliding traction with a 'fixed' Thomas's splint. The overhead frame (Thanet beam — Fig. 5.10) consists of one vertical upright attached to the centre of the head of the bed, and two vertical uprights attached to each side of the foot of the bed. These uprights are joined by two longitudinal horizontal bars. From a short transverse horizontal bar attached to the top of the single upright at the head of the bed, eight pulleys are suspended, four for each lower limb on each side of the upright (Fig. 5.10a). Four pulleys are attached to each longitudinal horizontal bar, two each at the level of the hip and the foot (Fig. 5.10b and 5.10c). A second transverse horizontal bar carrying two pulleys for the traction cords, joins the two uprights at the foot of the bed (Fig. 5.10c).

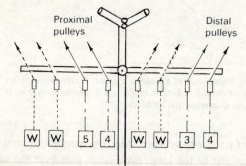

Fig. 5.10a   Thanet beam. Arrangement of pulleys, cords and weights on horizontal transverse bar at the head of the bed (weights in lbs).

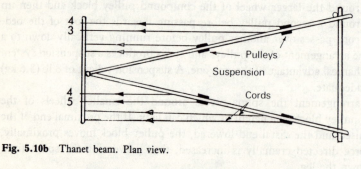

Fig. 5.10b   Thanet beam. Plan view.

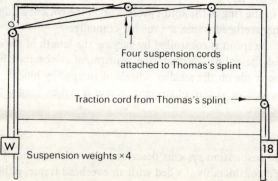

Fig. 5.10c   Thanet beam. Side view.

Eight cords with spring clips attached to each end are threaded through each of the eight pulleys suspended from the transverse bar at the head of the bed. Weights, which hang down behind the head of the bed, are attached to one end of each cord (Fig. 5.10a). The bed is thus ready to receive a patient.

Four suspension cords which must be at right angles to the splint are attached by the spring clips to loops of tape placed around the side bars of the Thomas's splint. The proximal loops are situated at the padded ring and the distal loops level with the foot. The weights attached to the two cords from the outer side bar of the splint are one pound (0.46 kg) heavier than those attached to the corresponding cords from the inner side bar (Fig. 5.11). In this way lateral rotation of the splint is controlled. Listed below are the suspension weights commonly used for adults. They have to be modified only rarely.

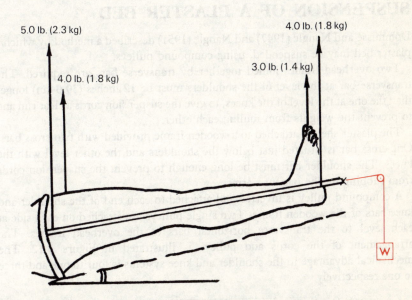

Fig. 5.11 Method 4. Suspension of Thomas's splint. Arrangement of suspension weights for sliding traction in a 'fixed' Thomas's splint, using a Thanet beam (Strange, 1972).

Proximal end of splint, outer side bar — 5 lb (2.3 kg)
inner side bar — 4 lb (1.8 kg)
Distal end of splint,   outer side bar — 4 lb (1.8 kg)
inner side bar — 3 lb (1.4 kg)

As sliding traction with a 'fixed' Thomas's splint is employed with this system of suspension, the suspension cords only have to suspend the splint; they do not have to maintain the position of the splint on the limb. The patient rapidly becomes very mobile, so mobile in fact that within two or three weeks of injury he is able to climb onto the overhead frame or stand by the side of his bed on his sound limb without any displacement of the fracture occurring.

USING SPRINGS

A Thomas's splint, to which a Böhler stirrup has been attached by brackets* at the centre of gravity of the limb near the knee, can be suspended from an overhead frame by a single spring incorporating a safety cord, and with a hook at each end (Denman, 1962). The spring passes upwards and cranially from the Böhler stirrup to the overhead frame.

Springs, of three different tensions, which measure 18 inches (46.0 cm) in length when lax and which stretch 6 inches (15.0 cm) in response to pulls of 15, 20, and 25 lb (6.8, 9.0, and 11.3 kg) respectively, are available.* Usually the spring of intermediate tension is used.

Rotation is controlled by varying the attachment of the spring to the Böhler stirrup.

SUSPENSION OF A PLASTER BED

Dommisse and Nangle (1947) and Nangle (1951) described a method by which a plaster bed may be suspended, using compound pulleys.

Two overhead frames joined together by transverse bars are required. The transverse bar at the level of the shoulders must be 12 inches (30.0 cm) longer than the one at the level of the knees, to give the suspension cords a clear run and to prevent the weights from fouling each other.

The plaster shell is attached to a wooden frame provided with two cross bars. One cross bar is situated just below the shoulders and the other level with the knees. The shoulder bar must be long enough to prevent the suspension cords from rubbing on the patient's arms.

A compound pulley is inverted and attached to each end of the shoulder and knee bars of the wooden frame. Two single pulleys are attached on each side at each level to the transverse horizontal bars of the overhead frames. The arrangement of the cords and pulleys is illustrated in Figure 5.12. The mechanical advantage in the shoulder and knee systems is four to one and three to one respectively.

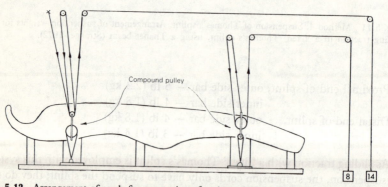

Compound pulley

Fig. 5.12 Arrangement of cords for suspension of a plaster bed. Note: arrows show direction in which cords run. The compound pulleys are attached to the wooden frame which supports the plaster bed, in opposite directions at the shoulders and knees.

* See Appendix.

The amount of weight required is determined for each patient. An average adult requires two 14 lb (6.3 kg) weights for the shoulder system and two 8 lb (3.6 kg) weights for the knee systm. The effect of these weights multiplied by the mechanical advantage (MA) of the pulley systems is as follows:

Shoulder bar system $2 \times (14 \text{ lb} \times 4) = 112 \text{ lb} (50.4 \text{ kg})$
Knee bar system $2 \times (8 \text{ lb} \times 3) = 48 \text{ lb} (21.6 \text{ kg})$

                                       Total lift = 160 lb (72.0 kg)

The counter-weights must be heavy enough to enable the patient and the plaster bed to be raised easily from the bed and to remain suspended.

SUSPENSION OF A PELVIC SLING

Minor pelvic fractures, for example isolated fractures of the pubic or ischial rami, are treated by rest in bed. When the pelvic ring has been opened out, a pelvic sling is used (Fig. 5.13). A pelvic sling is made from heavy canvas or Terylene 12 inches (30.0 cm) wide. It has hems at each side through which large diameter wooden or steel rods are passed. Cords pass from the pelvic sling over pulleys to weights.

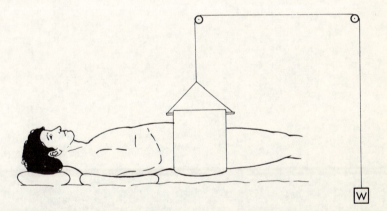

Fig. 5.13 Pelvic sling. The pelvic sling lies between the symphysis pubis and the posterior iliac crests. Sufficient weights are used to just lift the buttocks off the bed. There are pillows under the back and the head. The suspension cords are crossed if inward pressure is required.

APPLICATION OF A PELVIC SLING

— Place the pelvic sling under the buttocks, to lie between the symphysis pubis and the posterior iliac crests.
— Attach a cord to each end of the rods.

— Pass the cords over pulleys situated above the pelvic sling, and attach sufficient weights to lift the patient's buttocks just clear of the mattress.

— Place pillows under the patient's shoulders and back, to keep the patient horizontal and to avoid the sling's slipping up or down.

— To close the pelvic ring, cross the suspension cords to produce an inward pressure.

— Combine a pelvic sling with skeletal limb traction when there is upward displacement of one side of the pelvis.

REFERENCES

Bick, E.M. (1948) *Source Book of Orthopaedics*, p. 284. Baltimore: Williams & Wilkins.

Denman, E.E. (1962) Spring suspension for Thomas's splint. *British Medical Journal*, **ii**, 47.

Dommisse, G.F. & Nangle, E.J. (1947) The elimination of apparatus inertia in the treatment of fractures. *British Journal of Surgery*, **34**, 395.

Fisk, G.R. (1944) The fractured femoral shaft: new approach to the problem. *Lancet*, **i**, 659.

Nangle, E.J. (1951) *Instruments and Apparatus in Orthopaedic Surgery*, p. 89. Oxford: Blackwell.

Strange, F.G. St C. (1972) Personal communication.

6.

Spinal traction

Traction is required in the management of some conditions of the cervical, thoracic and lumbar spines.

In conditions of the cervical spine non-skeletal traction is obtained by applying a halter around the head, and skeletal traction by gaining purchase on the outer table of the skull with metal pins. A cord passes from the apparatus over a pulley, attached to the head of the bed, to a traction weight.

When traction is required for correction of deformities of the thoracic and lumbar spines, skeletal traction using the halo-pelvic method is employed.

HALTER OR NON-SKELETAL TRACTION

Halter traction is uncomfortable if it is applied continuously for more than a few hours. It is reserved usually for use in the treatment of cervical spondylosis as an out-patient.

A canvas or chamois leather head halter (Fig. 6.1)
This may be used. One part is placed under the chin and the other under the occiput. A metal spreader hooks onto the two side pieces to avoid lateral compression of the soft tissues when traction is applied. A cord from the metal spreader passes over a pulley fixed to the top of the bed and is attached to weights. The maximum weight which can be attached is 3–5 lb (1.4–2.3 kg). Pressure sores may develop under the chin or occiput, and in men beard growth may be troublesome. Eating is difficult.

The Crile head halter (Fig. 6.2)
This consists of a well-padded curved metal bar, resembling a horse collar, which is placed under the occiput. A padded forehead piece is attached by straps to the occipital piece. The chin is free. The maximum weight which can be attached is 3–5 lb (1.4–2.3 kg).
The head of the bed must be raised to provide counter-traction.

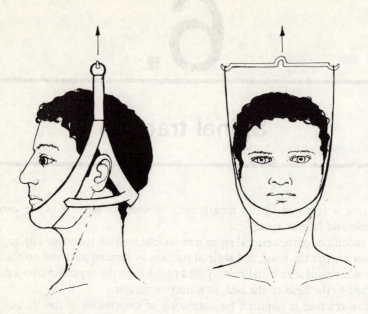

Fig. 6.1 Canvas head halter.

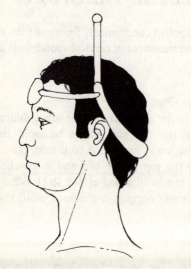
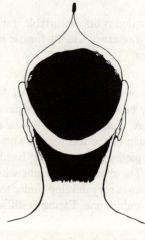

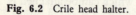

Fig. 6.2 Crile head halter.

SKULL OR SKELETAL TRACTION

Skull traction (Crutchfield, 1933) is achieved by gaining purchase on the outer table of the skull with metal pins. The metal pins are inserted under local anaesthesia. General anaesthesia is not used thus decreasing the risk of damage to the cervical spinal cord. Crutchfield or Cone (Barton) tongs or a halo splint may be used. A traction weight of 20–40 lb (9.1–18.2 kg) can be applied.

Skull traction is used commonly in the management of serious injuries to the cervical spine to reduce a dislocation or fracture-dislocation. In traction, the fracture or fracture-dislocation is under control and injury to the spinal cord is less likely to occur. Skull traction is used also to maintain the position of the cervical spine before and after operative fusion and for the treatment of cervical spondylosis with severe nerve root compression symptoms.

Crutchfield tongs (Fig. 6.3)
Crutchfield tongs fit into the parietal bones. A special drill point with a shoulder is used to enable an accurate depth of hole to be drilled (Crutchfield, 1954).

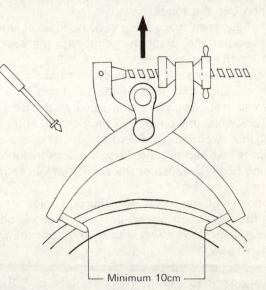

Fig. 6.3 Crutchfield tongs. Note that the points of the tongs are almost at right angles to the line of traction. The insert shows the special drill point with a shoulder which is used.

APPLICATION OF CRUTCHFIELD TONGS

— Sedate the patient.
— Shave the scalp locally. Excessive shaving is very distressing to the patient.
— Draw a line on the scalp, bisecting the skull from front to back (Fig. 6.4).

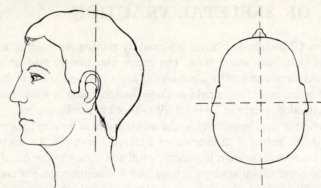

Fig. 6.4 Skull markings for positioning Crutchfield tongs. A vertical line through the tips of the mastoid processes crosses at right angles a second line bisecting the skull from front to back.

— Draw a second line joining the tips of the mastoid processes (the plane of the cervical articulations) which crosses the first line at right angles (Fig. 6.4).
— Fully open out the tongs.
— With the fully open tongs lying equally on each side of the antero-posterior line, press the points into the scalp making dimples on the second line.
— Infiltrate the area of the dimples down to and including the periosteum, with local anaesthetic solution.
— Make small stab wounds in the scalp at the dimples.
— Using the special drill point, drill through the outer table of the skull *in a direction parallel to the points of the tongs*. The drill point is inserted to a depth of 3 millimetres in children, care being taken because of the scanty diploic space, and 4 millimetres in adults.
— Fit the points of the tongs into the drill holes.
— Tighten the adjustment screw until a firm grip is obtained, *and repeat daily for the first 3 to 4 days,* and then tighten when necessary.
— Attach a traction cord to the two lugs.
— Attach a weight to the traction cord (see p. 80).
— Raise the head of the bed to provide counter-traction. Elevation must be increased as the traction weight is increased (Fig. 6.5).

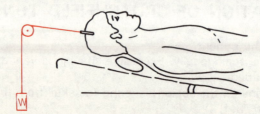

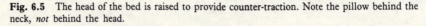

Fig. 6.5 The head of the bed is raised to provide counter-traction. Note the pillow behind the neck, *not* behind the head.

FAILURE OF THE PROCEDURE

Crutchfield (1954) stated that failure may be due to several factors.

1. The use of a faulty instrument. When opened out fully, the distance between the points should be 11 cm and certainly not less than 10 cm (Fig. 6.3).

2. Pins that are not long enough to prevent the arms of the tongs from crushing the scalp must not be used. In addition the pins must be set obliquely enough to the arms of the tongs, to ensure that they penetrate the diploe almost at right angles to the line of traction.

3. Placing the drill holes too close together in the skull.

4. Insufficient penetration of the skull.

5. Failure to keep the tongs tight.

Cone (Barton) tongs

The tongs were designed by Barton (Cone and Turner, 1937). A drill is not required for their insertion (Fig. 6.6). The threaded steel points are screwed into the parietal bones behind the ears.

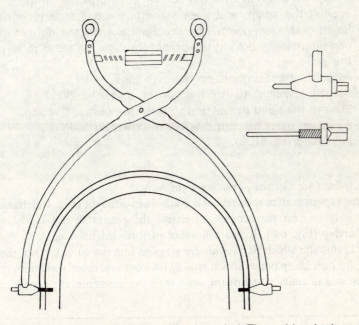

Fig. 6.6 Cone (Barton) tongs. No separate drilling is required. The special steel points are inserted into the conical ends of the tongs and tightened alternately.

APPLICATION OF CONE (BARTON) TONGS

— Sedate the patient.
— Draw a line up from the tip of the mastoid process to cross the sagittal plane at right angles (Fig. 6.7).

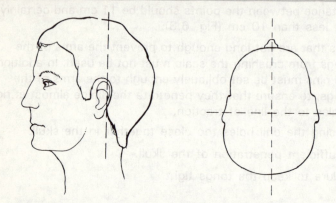

Fig. 6.7 Skull markings for Cone tongs. A vertical line through the mastoid processes, crosses at right angles a second line bisecting the skull from front to back.

— Shave the skull above and behind the ears.
— Open out the tongs sufficiently, and determine where the conical ends lie on the line drawn above.
— Infiltrate this area with local anaesthetic solution.
— Reapply the tongs with the conical ends pressed firmly against the scalp, and then make two small stab wounds.
— Insert both steel points into the conical ends and tighten each one alternately, driving the points through the outer table of the skull.
— Attach a traction cord to the two lugs.
— Attach a weight to the traction cord (see p. 80).
— Elevate the head of the bed to provide counter-traction. Elevation must be increased as the traction weight is increased (Fig. 6.5).

Halo splint (Ace Cervical Traction Equipment)*

The halo splint is an oval metal band available in different sizes, which arches up posteriorly to clear the occiput, to enable the patient to rest his head more comfortably (Fig. 6.8). It has a number of threaded holes at 2, 4, 8 and 10 o'clock, through which fixing pins are screwed into the outer table of the skull. The pins have sharp points which rapidly flare out into broad shoulders, creating a large area of contact against the skull with the minimum of penetration (Fig. 6.9).

*See Appendix.

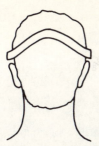
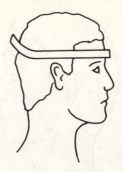
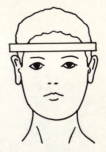

Fig. 6.8 The Ace halo splint.

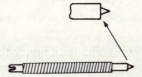

Fig. 6.9 The fixing pins used with the halo splint. Note the broad shoulders.

APPLICATION OF HALO SPLINT

— Choose a halo splint which will allow a clearance of $\frac{1}{2}$ inch (1.25 cm) on all sides of the head, when the splint is positioned with its *lower margin* lying just above the ears and about $\frac{1}{4}$ inch (6.0 mm) above the eyebrows.

— Autoclave the splint and pins.

— Lie the patient supine on an operating table with his head projecting over the end of the table. The patient's head is supported by an assistant on a 4 inch (10.0 cm) wide board placed under his head and back.

— Maintain control of the cervical spine by manual traction.

— Identify the *sites* for the four fixing pins — $\frac{3}{8}$ inch (1.0 cm) above the lateral one third of the eyebrows in the shallow grooves on the forehead between the supra-orbital ridges and frontal protuberances, and $\frac{3}{8}$ inch (1.0 cm) above the tops of the ears in line with the mastoid processes (Fig. 6.10).

— Shave the scalp for a distance of 2 inches (5.0 cm) around each pin site, and prepare the partly shaven scalp.

— Slip the halo splint over the skull with the raised portion posteriorly, and ask an assistant to hold it in the correct position.

— Advance the three *positioning* pins and plates so that the halo splint lies evenly around the skull.

— Infiltrate the sites of insertion of the *fixing* pins with 2 to 3 ml of 2% local anaesthetic solution.

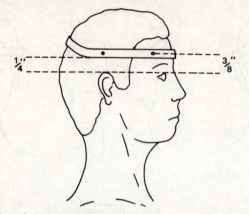

Fig. 6.10 Positioning of the halo splint, and the sites of insertion of the four fixing pins.

— Advance the four fixing pins until finger-tight. Incision of the scalp is not required.
— Using preset torque-limiting screwdrivers, further advance the pins in *diametrically opposed pairs at the same time,* to avoid side-to-side drifting of the halo splint, until slip occurs. The torque-limiting screwdrivers are preset to the following:

for children — 4.5 lb/inches — (5.1 kg/cm)
for adults — 6.0 lb/inches — (6.8 kg/cm)

— Remove the *positioning* screws.
— If traction is to be applied, fit the halo bail and cord (Fig. 6.11), or tie two cords to the halo splint, and attach the traction weight.
— Elevate the head of the bed to provide counter-traction.

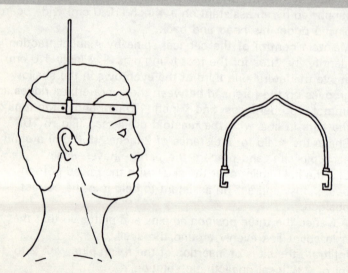

Fig. 6.11 The halo bail which is used if traction is to be applied to the halo splint.

DISLOCATION OR FRACTURE-DISLOCATION OF THE CERVICAL SPINE

The majority of serious injuries to the cervical spine result from forward flexion with or without an element of lateral flexion, and are therefore relatively stable in extension. Occasionally extension injuries occur, in which cases the spine is stable in flexion. In all injuries, rotation of the spine is dangerous.

It is not advisable to attempt a rapid reduction of a dislocation or fracture-dislocation of the cervical spine, as the spinal cord may be damaged if the initial pull is excessive.

AIMS OF TREATMENT

1. To avoid damage to the cervical cord.

2. To restore the antero-posterior diameter of the spinal canal.

3. To obtain complete reduction of the dislocation or fracture-dislocation. Although this is desirable it is not always possible. A decrease in the antero-posterior diameter of the spinal canal of less than 3 mm may be accepted (Rogers, 1957).

MANAGEMENT OF SKULL TRACTION

— Apply tongs or halo splint as described above.
— Apply minimum traction weight (see below).
— Take radiographs the following day.
— If reduction has not been obtained, gradually increase the traction weight. It is rarely necessary to more than double the minimum traction weight.
— When sufficient distraction has been obtained:
  1. Do not increase the traction weight further.
  2. Extend the cervical spine by placing a small rolled towel or sand-bag *under the neck* (*not* under the head as this will flex the cervical spine).
— When satisfactory alignment has been obtained, reduce the traction weight to 5–7 lb (2.3–3.2 kg) to maintain the corrected position, until the spine is stable. This takes 6–10 weeks.
— If a heavy traction weight is used initially, take radiographs at 15 minute intervals for at least one hour, or until it can be seen that the traction force is not too strong, and reduce the traction weight as soon as sufficient distraction has been obtained.

RECOMMENDED TRACTION WEIGHTS

For correction of deformity only (Crutchfield, 1954)

Table 6.1

Level	Minimum weight	Maximum weight
C1	5 lb (2.3 kg)	10 lb (4.5 kg)
C2	6 lb (2.7 kg)	10–12 lb (4.5–5.4 kg)
C3	8 lb (3.6 kg)	10–15 lb (4.5–6.7 kg)
C4	10 lb (4.5 kg)	15–20 lb (6.7–9.0 kg)
C5	12 lb (5.4 kg)	20–25 lb (9.0–11.3 kg)
C6	15 lb (6.7 kg)	20–30 lb (9.0–13.5 kg)
C7	18 lb (8.2 kg)	25–35 lb (11.3–15.8 kg)

These traction weights are approximately correct for the various levels of the cervical spine when the head of the patient's bed is raised not more than 20 degrees for the purpose of counter traction.

IMPORTANT: CHECK DAILY THAT

— The neurological examination of the patient has not changed.
— The tongs are applied firmly to the skull. If a halo splint is used, check daily for the first week, using a preset torque-limiting screwdriver (see above), that the fixing pins are tight. After the first week, the tightness of the fixing pins must be checked twice each week.
— The scalp wounds are not infected. If infection is present, the scalp wounds must be swabbed to discover the infecting organism and its antibiotic sensitivity. If Crutchfield or Cone tongs are used, they must be removed and another method of controlling the cervical spine substituted. If a halo splint is used, a new sterile pin is inserted through an adjacent hole, and tightened with a torque-limiting screwdriver *before* the infected pin is removed.
— The traction cord runs freely in the pulley and is not frayed.
— The traction weight is hanging free.
— The patient is neither being pulled up nor sliding down the bed. If he is, adjust the elevation of the head of the bed as necessary, to provide the correct amount of counter-traction.

COMPLICATIONS OF SKULL TRACTION

Crutchfield tongs may pull out of the skull. This results from failure to check that they are tight. They can be replaced under aseptic conditions, but it is better to substitute another method of controlling the cervical spine.

Crutchfield tongs may penetrate the inner table of the skull if they are over tightened. The patient complains of local pain. On examination one arm of the tongs is found to lie closer to the skull than the other. Tangential radiographs can be helpful. The tongs are removed, and another method of controlling the cervical spine is substituted. Subsequent complications rarely occur, unless there is associated infection of the pin site, as penetration of the inner table of the skull has occurred slowly.

Skeletal traction applied to the skull can give rise to complications which may be fatal — osteomyelitis of the skull, extradural haematoma, extradural abscess, subdural abscess, cerebral abscess (Weisl, 1971).

These complications may be heralded by pyrexia and headaches, and progress to fits, hemiplegia and coma. Examination of the cerebrospinal fluid and cerebral angiography may be normal. In the presence of osteomyelitis of the skull, radiographic examination may show radiolucent areas at the site of insertion of the pins.

If infection is suspected, the scalp wounds must be swabbed to discover the infecting organism and its antibiotic sensitivity, so that the appropriate antibiotic can be given. Skull traction must be discontinued and another method of controlling the cervical spine substituted.

HALO-BODY ORTHOSIS

The halo-body orthosis was introduced originally in 1959 by Perry and Nickel, in the management of paralytic deformities of the cervical and thoracic spines. Its application was described in detail by Thompson (1962), Nickel et al (1968) and Stewart (1975). It consisted of a halo splint, attached to the skull by four screws, which was suspended from a jointed adjustable overhead frame incorporated in a plaster-of-Paris jacket. The jacket extended from the shoulders to the iliac crests, purchase on the body being obtained by the close moulding of the jacket around the iliac crests. The neck was free of plaster (Fig. 6.12).

This apparatus was cumbersome and made it difficult for patients to pass through doorways or to travel in private or public transport. Houtkin and Levine (1972) made the apparatus less bulky. They eliminated the projecting overhead frame and attached the halo to a plaster-of-Paris jacket by two adjustable yokes. With further development, the plaster jacket has been replaced by a premoulded, padded polyethylene vest. A number of different complete assemblies are now available commercially (Ace Orthopaedic).*

Halo vest
The padded polyethylene vest consists of two halves, anterior and posterior, which are strapped together over the shoulders and around the lower chest. Attached to each half of the vest are two metal uprights. These are connected

*See Appendix.

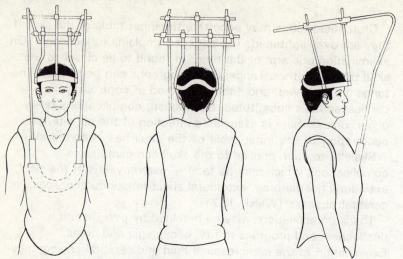

Fig. 6.12 The original halo-body orthosis, with the halo suspended from an overhead frame which was incorporated in a plaster jacket.

together on each side of the head by short horizontal metal bars, to which the halo splint is attached (Fig. 6.13). The position of the head can be adjusted in all directions, until the optimum position is obtained.

The development of the less cumbersome halo-body orthosis, which restricts, by at least 95%, all movements in the cervical spine (Johnson et al, 1977), has resulted in a reduction in the length of time a patient may have to stay in hospital after a serious injury to his cervical spine. The halo-body orthosis can be applied within a few days of a satisfactory reduction of a dislocation or a fracture-dislocation of the cervical spine having been obtained.

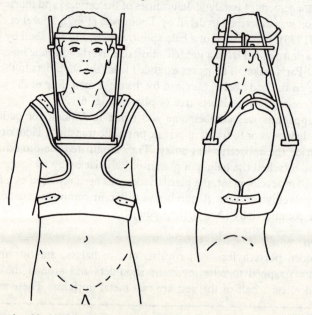

Fig. 6.13 The Ace Mark III halo-body orthosis. Compare this with Fig. 6.12.

APPLICATION OF THE HALO-BODY
ORTHOSIS (Ace Orthopaedic)*

— Apply the halo splint (see above).
— Measure the circumference of the patient's chest at the level of the xiphisternum, and choose the correct size of halo vest.
— Separate the anterior and posterior halves of the halo vest, but leave the metal bars, which cross over the shoulders, attached to the posterior half of the vest.
— Rotate the metal bar laterally.
— While maintaining the position of the patient's neck, gently raise the patient's shoulders and upper trunk sufficiently to slide the posterior half of the halo vest under the patient.
— Make sure that the posterior half of the vest is positioned as low as possible.
— Rotate the metal bars medially so that they lie directly over the shoulders.
— Place the anterior half of the vest in position.
— Secure the two halves of the vest together by fastening all the straps firmly.
— Assemble the metal framework. The exact details of assembly will depend upon which of the three different orthoses is used (Low Profile Halo; Mark II Halo; Mark III Halo).
— Take radiographs to check the position of the cervical vertebrae.
— Adjust the position of the head as necessary until the optimum position is obtained.
— Check that all locking nuts on the metal framework are tight.

HALO-PELVIC TRACTION

Halo-pelvic traction (Fig. 6.14) consists of a halo splint connected, by four vertical spring-loaded distraction rods, to a steel pelvic hoop. The pelvic hoop in turn is attached to two long threaded steel rods, each of which passes through one wing of the ilium (Dewald and Ray, 1970; O'Brien et al, 1971).

This form of skeletal traction may be used to immobilize the spine or to slowly correct or reduce deformities of the spine, such as occur in scoliosis and tuberculosis, before spinal fusion is carried out. The halo-pelvic apparatus remains in place during the operation and for a variable period of time afterwards. Patients in halo-pelvic traction may remain ambulant.

The halo splint is basically similar to that described above except that posteriorly the band does not arch upwards to clear the occipital area, and it is drilled and tapped around its perimeter to accept screws for the attachment of the four spring-loaded distraction rods.

*See Appendix.

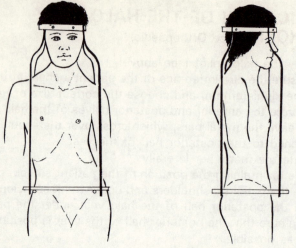

Fig. 6.14 Halo-pelvic traction.

Each threaded rod transfixes one wing of the ilium, passing through the thickest portion of the pelvis (Fig. 6.15), from the tubercle of the iliac crest to the posterior superior iliac spine on the same side.

The pelvic hoop, which must be of large enough diameter to allow a gap of 1–$1\frac{1}{2}$ inches (2.5–3.8 cm) between the patient's skin and the hoop, is attached to the threaded rods by four universal clamps. Superiorly the spring-loaded distraction bars are attached to the halo splint. Inferiorly they pass through four universal clamps, different from those which clamp the pelvic hoop to the threaded rods, on the pelvic hoop. Locking nuts are placed on each distraction rod, one above and one below the clamp. By adjusting the position of these locking nuts, the effective length of the distraction rods can be increased, thus increasing the distance between the halo splint and the pelvic hoop and thereby exerting a distraction force upon the spine.

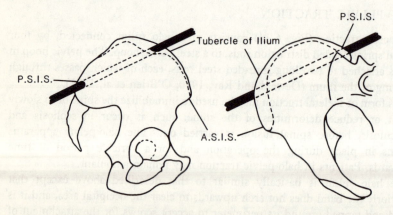

Lateral Aspect of Pelvis   Hemi Pelvis Seen From Above

Fig. 6.15 Halo-pelvic traction. Each threaded rod transfixes one wing of the ilium, passing from the tubercle of the iliac crest to the posterior superior iliac spine (PSIS) on the same side.

APPLICATION OF HALO-PELVIC TRACTION

Halo-pelvic traction may be applied under endotracheal anaesthesia or after the administration of Ketamine Hydrochloride* (Ketalar, Parke-Davis).

1. Halo splint

Under full aseptic conditions, apply the halo splint as described above.

2. Pelvic rods and hoop

— Mount a threaded rod in a hand brace.
— Make a small stab wound opposite the tubercle of the ilium (Ransford and Manning, 1978), which may be as much as 2 inches (5.0 cm) superior and posterior to the anterior superior iliac spine. The tubercle of the ilium can be palpated easily, as the subcutaneous iliac crest is widest at this point. In fat patients, where palpation can be difficult, make an incision just posterior to the summit of the iliac crest large enough to allow a finger to pass downwards inside the inner table of the ilium (Ransford and Manning, 1978).
— Position the drilling jig (Cass and Dwyer, 1969). Place the posterior end of the jig over the posterior superior iliac spine, and then insert the anterior end of the jig through the stab wound on the same side until it impinges on the pelvis opposite the tubercle of the ilium. Tighten the jig. The use of the jig ensures the correct positioning of the threaded rods (Fig. 6.15).
— Check the position of the jig by pushing a Steinmann pin through the anterior part of the jig into the ilium.
— Insert the mounted threaded rod into the jig and drill it through the wing of the ilium in an antero-posterior direction, removing the jig when the point of the rod emerges posteriorly from the bony pelvis.
— Continue drilling until about 6 inches (15.0 cm) projects posteriorly.
— Cut off the sharp points of the pelvic rods.
— Insert the second rod through the opposite wing of the ilium in the same manner.
— Apply small dry dressings around the entry and exit wounds.
— Clamp the pelvic hoop to the threaded rods, arranging the hoop to lie evenly around the pelvis. The pelvic hoop will lie obliquely. Keeping the anterior part of the hoop high allows the patient to sit more comfortably.

---

*See Appendix.

— Remove the lengths of the threaded rods projecting beyond the pelvic hoop by cutting them with heavy-duty bolt cutters.
— Return the patient to the ward.

3. **Distraction rods** (Fig. 6.16)

Delay fitting the distraction rods for 48 hours. This allows easier abdominal examination in the event of peritoneal penetration by the pelvic rods (see below, Ransford and Manning, 1978).

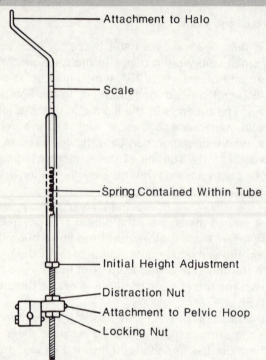

Attachment to Halo

Scale

Spring Contained Within Tube

Initial Height Adjustment

Distraction Nut

Attachment to Pelvic Hoop

Locking Nut

Fig. 6.16 Spring-loaded distraction rod for halo-pelvic traction.

If the spine is unstable because of the presence of a fracture or fracture-dislocation, apply traction to the halo splint to immobilise the spine until the distraction rods are fitted.
— Sit the patient comfortably on a stool.
— Apply traction to the halo splint so that the patient sits erect with his buttocks almost raised from the stool.
— Ensure that the cervical spine is neither flexed nor extended.
— Measure the exact distance between the halo and the pelvic hoop.
— Adjust the length of each distraction rod to the above measurements to achieve a zero reading on the fixed scale.

— Position the second set of four universal clamps on the pelvic hoop so that they lie at the corners of a square, two antero-laterally and two postero-laterally.

— Insert the lower threaded end of each distraction rod through one of the universal clamps.

— Select suitable holes on the halo splint at approximately 2, 4, 8 and 10 o'clock, and attach the upper end of each distraction rod to the halo splint.

— Carefully adjust the position of the universal clamps on the pelvic hoop so that the distraction rods lie evenly disposed on each side of the patient and do not interfere with movement of the upper limbs. The distraction rods may have to be contoured, when there is a large rib hump or pelvic obliquity, to avoid pressure on the skin.

— Release the traction on the halo splint.

— Adjust the length of the distraction rods as necessary until the previous recorded halo-hoop distance is reached. This may compress the spring giving an initial reading on the fixed scales.

— Note the reading on the fixed scales.

— If the position of the distraction rods is satisfactory, tighten all screws and nuts on the halo splint, distraction rods, and pelvic hoop with a spanner, Allan key or screwdriver. Remember that the cranial screws on the halo splint must be tightened only with a torque-limiting screwdriver.

— Return the patient to the ward.

MANAGEMENT OF HALO-PELVIC TRACTION

— Daily after the insertion of the pelvic rods, examine the abdomen for the development of any abdominal complications (see below).

— Every patient in halo-pelvic traction must be examined daily, especially while distraction is being carried out, for the presence of any neurological complications (see below).

— Examine the scalp wounds daily for the presence of infection (see under skull traction).

— Daily for the first week and then twice weekly, check the tightness of the cranial screws (see under skull traction).

— Examine the wounds around the pelvic rods at regular intervals for the presence of infection. If infection is present, swab the wound to determine the infecting organism and its antibiotic sensitivity. Infection at these sites usually responds rapidly to regular cleansing with an antibacterial solution and systemic antibiotics.

— Ask the patient if he feels pain around the pelvic rods. Pain may be caused by infection or loosening of the rods.

— Check that all the screws and nuts on the pelvic hoop and distraction rods are tight. This must be carried out twice each week until the apparatus is removed.

— Wash the patient's hair once or twice each week.

— Distraction. Ransford and Manning (1975) perform preliminary myelography in all cases where there is suspicion of diastematomyelia and in all cases with an osteogenic aetiology.

Distraction is commenced four days after the spring-loaded distraction rods have been attached.

Each day, distract all four rods by one turn of the distraction nut (1.25 mm, equivalent to a force of 0.25 kg per rod — this will vary according to the strength of the distraction spring used in the rods). Continue distraction until the reading on the fixed scale is between 16 and 18 kilograms, or until the patient suffers painful spasms of the neck muscles, or neurological complications develop (see below). A total of 18 kilograms distraction force is never exceeded (Ransford and Manning, 1975).

If neurological complications occur, immediately reduce the distraction force.

COMPLICATIONS OF HALO-PELVIC TRACTION

(See also complications of skull traction, p. 80.)

A. Cranial screws

1. Superficial infection around the cranial screws.
2. Cerebral abscess (Victor et al, 1973).
3. Loosening of the cranial screws.
4. Pain when the cranial screws are tightened. This may occur from the surrounding skin puckering up circumferentially.
5. Penetration of the inner table of the skull by the cranial screws (Ransford and Manning, 1975). This is diagnosed by the failure of a screw to tighten after minimal screwing, and is confirmed radiographically by tangential views. The screw is removed and a new screw inserted in a nearby hole under local anaesthesia and full aseptic precautions. Prophylactic systemic antibiotics are given.

B. Pelvic rods

1. Vague aches and pains are sometimes felt around the hips and can extend down the thigh or into the buttock. These symptoms usually subside within a few days but if they are severe enough to cause difficulty in walking without assistance they can be relieved by removing the pelvic rods (O'Brien et al, 1971).
2. Peritoneal penetration by a pelvic rod with or without bowel damage. This is most likely to occur if the anterior entry point is close to the anterior superior iliac spine. To avoid peritoneal penetration the anterior entry point must be opposite the tubercle of the ilium, which may be 2 inches (5.0 cm) superior and posterior to the anterior superior iliac spine (Ransford and Manning, 1978).
3. Superficial infection. This is more common around the anterior entry holes. If it occurs a swab is taken for culture and antibiotic sensitivity, and the appropriate systemic antibiotic is given. In the presence of severe infection the pelvic rod is removed.
4. Loosening.
5. Hip contracture from ilio-psoas fibrosis (Kalamchi et al, 1976).

C. Neurological

These are less likely to occur when spring-loaded distraction rods are used (Ransford and Manning, 1975). They may result from traction lesions of peripheral or cranial nerves or the spinal cord. They may be temporary or permanent.

Abducent nerve palsy — the patient is unable to move the affected eye in an outward direction. Contraction of the internal rectus muscle eventually leads to internal strabismus and diplopia.

Glosso-pharyngeal nerve palsy — the patient complains of difficulty in swallowing and may choke. There is loss of sensation to touch and taste over the posterior third of the tongue (Manning, 1972).

Recurrent laryngeal nerve palsy — hoarseness.

Hypoglossal nerve palsy — on protrusion, the tongue deviates to the affected side.

Brachial plexus palsy — either the upper or lower or all of the components of the brachial plexus (C5, C6, C7, C8 and T1) may be involved.

Spinal cord — paraplegia. Preliminary myelography is advisable in all cases where there is suspicion of diastematomyelia or osteogenic aetiology (Ransford and Manning, 1975).

When any of the above neurological complications occur, distraction must be discontinued immediately.

Paraesthesiae in the distribution of the lateral cutaneous nerve of the thigh may occur following insertion of the pelvic rods. It settles in one to two weeks without any specific measures being taken.

D. General

1. Death from respiratory insufficiency.
2. Osteoporosis of the vertebrae.
3. Cervical subluxation C1 on C2. This results from the incorrect application of the appliance with the cervical spine in flexion (Kalamchi et al, 1976).
4. Avascular necrosis of the proximal pole of the odontoid process (Morton and Malins, 1971).
5. Cervical spondylosis has been suggested as a long term complication (O'Brien et al, 1973; Kalamchi et al, 1976).
6. Enuresis may reappear if there has been a history of it in the past. Imipramine in appropriate dosage may be given.

REFERENCES

Cass, C.A.& Dwyer, A.F. (1969) A drilling jig for arthrodesis of the hip. *Journal of Bone and Joint Surgery*, **51-B**, 135.
Cone, W. & Turner, W.G. (1937) The treatment of fracture-dislocation of the cervical vertebrae by skeletal traction and fusion. *Journal of Bone and Joint Surgery*, **19**, 584.
Crutchfield, W.G. (1933) Skeletal traction for dislocation of the cervical spine. Report of a case. *Southern Surgeon*, **2**, 156.
Crutchfield, W.G. (1954) Skeletal traction in treatment of injuries to the cervical spine. *Journal of the American Medical Association*, **155**, 29.
Dewald, R.L. & Ray, R.D. (1970) Skeletal traction for the treatment of severe scoliosis. *Journal of Bone and Joint Surgery*, **52-A**, 233.
Houtkin, S. & Levine, D.B. (1972) The halo yoke. A simplified device for attachment of the halo to a body cast. *Journal of Bone and Joint Surgery*, **54-A**, 881.
Johnson, R.M., Hart, D.L., Simmons, E.F., Rambsy, G.R. & Southwick, W.O. (1977) Cervical orthoses. A study comparing their effectiveness in restricting motion in normal subjects. *Journal of Bone and Joint Surgery*, **59-A**, 332.
Kalamchi, A., Yau, A.C.M.C., O'Brien, J.P. & Hodgson, A.R. (1976) Halo-pelvic distraction apparatus. *Journal of Bone and Joint Surgery*, **58-A**, 1119.
Manning, C.W.S.F. (1972) Personal communication.
Morton, J. & Malins, P. (1971) The correction of spinal deformities by halo-pelvic traction. *Physiotherapy*, **57**, 576.
Nickel, V.L., Perry, J., Garrett, A. & Heppenstall, M. (1968) The halo; a spinal skeletal traction fixation device. *Journal of Bone and Joint Surgery*, **50-A**, 1400.
O'Brien, J.P., Yau, A.C.M.C., Smith, T.K. & Hodgson, A.R. (1971) Halo-pelvic traction. A preliminary report on a method of external skeletal fixation for correcting deformities and maintaining fixation of the spine. *Journal of Bone and Joint Surgery*, **53-B**, 217.
O'Brien, J.P., Yau, A.C.M.C. & Hodgson, A.R. (1973) Halo-pelvic traction: a technique for severe spinal deformity. *Clinical Orthopaedics and Related Research*, **93**, 179.
Perry, J. & Nickel, V.L. (1959) Total cervical fusion for neck paralysis. *Journal of Bone and Joint Surgery*, **41-A**, 37.

Ransford, A.O. & Manning, C.W.S.F. (1975) Complications of halo-pelvic distraction for scoliosis. *Journal of Bone and Joint Surgery*, **57-B,** 131.

Ransford, A.O. & Manning, C.W.S.F. (1978) Halo-pelvic apparatus: Peritoneal penetration by pelvic pins. *Journal of Bone and Joint Surgery*, **60-B,** 404.

Rogers, W.A. (1957) Fracture and dislocation of the cervical spine. An end-result study. *Journal of Bone and Joint Surgery*, **39-A,** 341.

Stewart, J.D.M. (1975) *Traction and Orthopaedic Appliances*, pp. 65–68, 1st edn. Edinburgh: Churchill Livingstone.

Thompson, H. (1962) The halo traction apparatus. *Journal of Bone and Joint Surgery*, **44-B,** 655.

Victor, D.I., Bresnan, M.J. & Keller, R.B. (1973) Brain abscess complicating the use of halo traction. *Journal of Bone and Joint Surgery*, **55-A,** 635.

Weisl, H. (1971) Unusual complications of skull caliper traction. *Journal of Bone and Joint Surgery*, **54-B,** 143.

7.

Splinting for congenital dislocation of the hip

The detection of the unstable hip as soon as possible after birth, and its prompt treatment, are vital. There is no direct evidence that every unstable hip at birth will, if untreated, become a dislocated hip, but if every hip that is found to be unstable at birth is treated, established dislocation of the hip virtually disappears (Rosen, 1962).

Unstable hips at birth are diagnosed clinically. All doctors who work with the new-born must know how to detect an unstable hip. Barlow (1962) found only 159 unstable hips in 9000 births, an incidence of 18 per 1000 (as opposed to 1.5 per 1000 for the incidence of established dislocation of the hip in Western Europe). This means that many normal hips will be examined before an unstable hip is found.

CLINICAL TESTS FOR UNSTABLE HIPS

BARLOW'S TEST (1962)

This test must be carried out within two to three days of birth, in a warm room and preferably after the child has been fed, when he will be relaxed and contented. The examiner's hands must be warm. The test is carried out in two stages.

STAGE ONE

— Remove the child's nappy.
— Place the child supine on a warm firm surface with its legs pointing towards you.
— Hold the knees fully flexed, with the flexed legs in the palms of your hands, and with the middle finger of each hand on the greater trochanter and the thumb on the inner aspect of the thigh opposite the lesser trochanter (Fig. 7.1).
— Flex the hips to a right angle and abduct them to 45 degrees.
— Press forwards *in turn* with the middle finger of each hand on the greater trochanter and attempt to lift the femoral head into the acetabulum.

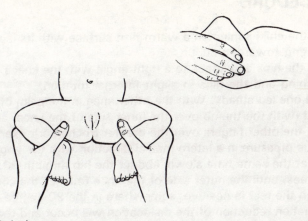

Fig. 7.1 Barlow's test.

The test is positive when the joint is dislocated and the femoral head returns to the acetabulum with a palpable and often audible clunk or jerk. The clunk or jerk is due to the femoral head snapping back over the posterior rim of the acetabulum into the socket. This must not be confused with ligamentous clicking, which can often be elicited from a baby's normal hip.

STAGE TWO

— Continue to hold the lower limbs as described above.
— Press backwards *in turn* with each thumb on the inner side of the thigh. If the femoral head slips backwards onto the posterior lip of the acetabulum or actually dislocates, the hip is unstable.
— In doubtful cases, firmly hold the pelvis with one hand, with the thumb on the pubis and the fingers under the sacrum, while performing the above test on one hip with the opposite hand.
— Examine the second hip in the same way.

This test is reliable and can be used up to the age of six months, by which time the femora have become so long that it is difficult to reach the greater trochanters with the tips of the middle fingers.

ORTOLANI'S TEST

This test was described by Ortolani in 1948 for use in children between three and nine months old. It is not entirely satisfactory in the new-born (Barlow, 1962).

PROCEDURE

— Lay the child supine on a warm firm surface with its legs
  pointing towards you.
— Flex the hips and knees to a right angle with the knees
  touching and the hips in slight internal rotation.
— Hold one leg steady. With the other knee in the palm of your
  hand (with the thumb over the inner side of the knee, and
  with the other fingers over the greater trochanter), exert
  gentle pressure in a latero-medial direction with the fingers
  and at the same time slowly abduct the hip through 90
  degrees, until the outer side of the knee touches the couch.
  When the test is positive, somewhere in the 90 degree arc of
  abduction reduction of the dislocation will occur and the head
  of the femur will slip into the acetabulum with a visible and
  palpable movement — a clunk or jerk.

The tests described above are generally reliable, but they may be misleading in
certain situations. When limited abduction of a hip is present due to contraction
of its adductor muscles, a clunk may not be elicited. However the presence of
limitation of abduction itself may indicate dislocation of that hip. 'Clicks' as
opposed to clunks or jerks can often be elicited on manipulation of the normal
hips of the new-born.

The incidence of unstable hips decreases in the first few weeks after birth.
Nelson (1966) found, on the examination of 866 live births, an incidence of 15.9
per cent soon after birth which fell to 7 per cent seven to ten days after birth, and
to 0.35 per cent at three weeks. The decrease in the incidence of unstable hips in
the weeks immediately after birth gives rise to some controversy as to whether an
unstable hip at birth should be treated immediately or whether only those which
are still unstable some weeks after birth should be treated. It is not within the
scope of this book to discuss the indications for treatment. Generally, however, it
is better to err on the side of over-treatment, as long as the treatment is carried
out correctly, and as long as the treatment does not give rise to any
complications.

RADIOGRAPHIC EXAMINATION

Ossification in the capital epiphysis of the femur is not present at birth and
therefore the capital epiphysis cannot be demonstrated radiologically. This
makes the radiographic identification of a dislocated hip in the young child
difficult. However, the ossific nucleus of the femoral head can be seen
radiographically in 78 per cent of normal hips at six months of age and in 99 per
cent at one year (Wynne-Davies, 1970).

UNDER SIX MONTHS OF AGE

Andrén and von Rosen (1958) described a technique for use in this age group in which an antero-posterior radiograph is taken with the child supine and with both lower limbs in full medial rotation and 45 degrees of abduction.

When the head of the femur is dislocated, the upward prolongation of the long axis of the shaft of the femur points towards the anterior superior iliac spine and crosses the midline in the lower lumbar region of the spine (Fig. 7.2). When the hip is not dislocated, the upward prolongation of the long axis of the shaft of the femur points towards the lateral margin of the acetabulum and crosses the posterior part of the pelvis in the region of the sacro-iliac joint (Fig. 7.2).

As a dislocated hip may reduce with abduction, it is possible to obtain a false negative result with this technique.

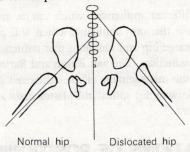

Normal hip   Dislocated hip

Fig. 7.2 Von Rosen radiograph of the hips; an antero-posterior radiograph with the lower limbs in full medial rotation and 45° abduction in a child under six months.

OVER SIX MONTHS OF AGE

Once the ossific nucleus of the femoral head is present, standard antero-posterior radiographs of the pelvis and hips, with the legs together and in neutral rotation, can be used.

In a normal hip, the ossific nucleus of the femoral head lies below the horizontal line (of Hilgenreiner) passing through the tri-radiate cartilages of the acetabula, and medial to the vertical line (of Perkins) passing through the outer lip of the acetabulum, perpendicular to the above horizontal line (Fig. 7.3).

When the head of the femur is dislocated, the ossific nucleus of the head tends to lie lateral to the vertical line and above the horizontal line (Fig. 7.3).

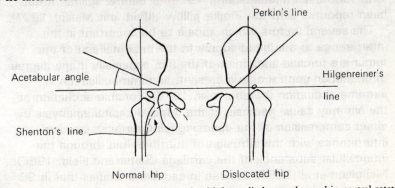

Perkin's line

Acetabular angle

Hilgenreiner's line

Shenton's line

Normal hip   Dislocated hip

Fig. 7.3 Standard antero-posterior radiograph with lower limbs together and in neutral rotation in a child over six months.

FURTHER RADIOGRAPHIC FINDINGS IN CONGENITAL
DISLOCATION OF THE HIP (Fig. 7.3)

The ossific nucleus of the dislocated hip is smaller, or its appearance is delayed,
compared with the normal side.

The angle between the horizontal line of Hilgenreiner and the line of the
acetabular roof (acetabular angle or index) is greater than 35 degrees.

Shenton's line is broken.

APPLIANCES AND PLASTER CASTS USED TO OBTAIN AND MAINTAIN THE REDUCTION OF A DISLOCATED HIP

Five of the many different appliances which can be used, are described below.
The Pavlik harness is the only appliance which will promote the spontaneous
reduction of a dislocated hip and maintain that reduction. The other appliances
will only maintain reduction. The von Rosen and Barlow splints and the Frejka
pillow are used in the management of the dislocated hip diagnosed soon after
birth. The Denis Browne hip splint and plaster casts are used only in the later
stages of management.

COMPLICATIONS OF POSITIONING OF THE HIPS

Avascular necrosis of the femoral capital epiphysis and
abnormalities of growth of the upper end of the femur can
develop in children who are being treated for congenital
dislocation of the hip. These changes can occur on both the
normal and abnormal sides, and as they do not occur in
untreated dislocations they probably are related to treatment
(Gore, 1974), and result from interference to the blood supply
to the proximal end of the femur.

Interference to this blood supply is more likely to occur with
immobilisation in plaster casts (Allen, 1962; Gore, 1974) than
with von Rosen (Fredensborg, 1976) or Barlow splints. It has
been reported with the Frejka pillow (Ilfeld and Makin, 1977).

The several factors which appear to be important in the
interference to the blood supply to the proximal end of the
femur are forcible abduction of the hip, especially if any degree
of adduction contracture is present, and immobilisation in
extreme abduction (Westin et al, 1976). Forcible abduction of
the hip may cause necrosis of the femoral capital epiphysis by
direct compression of the opposing joint surfaces causing
interference with the diffusion of nutritive fluid through the
intercellular substance of the cartilage (Salter and Field, 1960).
Nicholson et al (1954) showed in cadaveric studies that in 90
degrees of abduction, the blood supply to the femoral head is

seriously impaired. Ogden and Southwick (1973) and Ogden (1974) carried out injection and dissection studies of hips from stillborn and infant cadavera. They demonstrated that with abduction of the hip beyond 45 degrees, the developing acetabular rim fitted tightly into the intra-epiphyseal groove between the femoral head and the greater trochanter. This intra-epiphyseal groove carries the major blood supply to the femoral head. In abduction beyond 45 degrees, the medial femoral circumflex artery, from which the intra-epiphyseal circulation was usually derived, was stretched and compressed over and between the iliopsoas and adductor muscles.

In applying any of the following splints, including the Pavlik harness and Frejka pillow, or plaster casts, it is very important that neither the dislocated hip is forcibly reduced, nor the normal or abnormal hip is held rigidly in abduction beyond 45 degrees. It is important to allow a controlled range of movement to preserve the blood supply to the upper end of the femur.

PAVLIK HARNESS

Arnold Pavlik, a Czechoslovakian orthopaedic surgeon, introduced his method of treatment of congenital dislocation of the hip in 1944 (Erlacher, 1962). This method promotes spontaneous reduction of the dislocated hip by positioning the hip in flexion while allowing free abduction, thus minimising the risk of avascular necrosis. It is of particular use in children during the first six months of life.

The Pavlik harness * (Fig. 7.4) consists of an adjustable band encircling the lower chest. To this are attached a pair of shoulder straps, which cross posteriorly and a pair of stirrups which embrace the legs down to the heels. The stirrups are suspended from the encircling chest band by two adjustable straps, one passing anterior to and the other posterior to the lower limb. The harness allows active movement in all directions except extension, and adduction across the midline. Nappies can be changed easily and independently of the harness; the child's clothes fit easily over the harness; and the child can lie prone or supine.

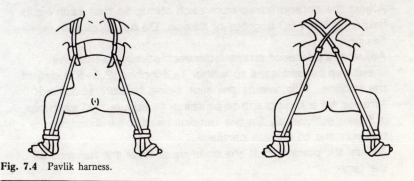

Fig. 7.4 Pavlik harness.

*See Appendix.

POINTS TO BE REMEMBERED WHEN USING A PAVLIK HARNESS (Ramsey et al, 1976)

1. Force must not be used when attempting reduction of the hip. The adductor muscles, if tight initially, will gradually and spontaneously stretch.
2. The position of the hip in flexion/abduction must be confirmed radiographically at the time of application to ensure that it is correct.
3. The hips must be flexed in excess of 90 degrees. Flexion must never be forced. Further spontaneous flexion must be able to occur from the final position. Inadequate flexion is the most common cause of failure of reduction of the hip. Because of the normal degree of valgus of the femoral head and neck, the femoral head will not be directed towards the tri-radiate cartilage, unless the hip is flexed at least 90 degrees. If the hip is flexed to less than 90 degrees, the femoral head will be directed towards the superior part of the acetabulum.
4. The posterior straps attaching the leg stirrups to the encircling band must not be tight, in order to avoid forcing abduction. These straps must be loose enough to allow the knees to be adducted to within 1–2 inches (2.5–5.0 cm) of the midline.
5. The stability of the femoral head must be assessed frequently during the initial stages of treatment.

APPLICATION OF THE PAVLIK HARNESS
(Fig. 7.4)

— Lie the child supine.
— Apply the harness, and adjust the shoulder straps to allow the encircling band to fit snugly around the lower chest.
— Fit the stirrups around the legs.
— Adjust the anterior strap from each stirrup so that each hip is held in at least 90 degrees of flexion. Do not force full flexion.
— Adjust the posterior straps from each stirrup so that the knees can be adducted to within 1–2 inches (2.5–5.0 cm) of the midline. This avoids the hips being forcibly abducted.
— Arrange for a radiograph to be taken to ensure that each hip is flexed sufficiently for the femoral head to be directed towards the tri-radiate cartilage.
— Advise the parents that the child must wear the harness all the time.

— Examine the harness and the dislocated hip regularly. The first examination is carried out after two days and then at weekly intervals until the hip becomes clinically stable.
— When the hip is clinically stable, remove the harness for two hours each day, increasing the time the child is out of the harness by 2–4 hours every two weeks as long as an antero-posterior radiograph is consistent with the hip being reduced, the acetabular angle is stable or increasing, and the femoral capital epiphysis, if present, is enlarging.

VON ROSEN SPLINT (Rosen, 1956)

The von Rosen splint (Fig. 7.5) is H-shaped, the crossbar of the H being extended on each side. It is cut from malleable aluminium sheeting, padded and covered with latex rubber or plastic, the latter being less irritating to the skin of some children. Three sizes of splint are available.

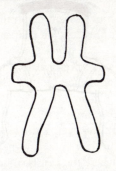
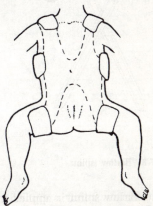

Fig. 7.5   Von Rosen splint.

APPLICATION OF THE VON ROSEN SPLINT
(Fig. 7.5)

— Choose a splint of adequate size.
— Place the child supine on the splint.
— Mould the upper limbs of the splint over the shoulders, taking care that they do not press on the sides of the child's neck, or on its nipples.
— Mould the short central limbs of the splint around the child's trunk.
— Reduce the hip and maintain the reduction by moulding the lower limbs of the splint up and around the child's thighs, so that the hips are held loosely in 90 degrees of flexion and not more than 45 degrees of abduction. It must be possible to obtain this position easily without using force.

— Check that the child and especially the lower limbs do not come out of the splint when the child moves. Check also that the limbs are not held rigidly, as some movement of the limbs within the splint is essential.

BARLOW SPLINT (Barlow, 1962)

The Barlow splint (Fig. 7.6) consists of two strips of malleable aluminium 1 inch wide and 22 inches long (2.5 cm by 55 cm) held together by a single rivet 9 inches (22.5 cm) below the top end. The aluminium strips are padded on one side with felt, are covered with soft leather and are provided with a canvas strap which can be passed through slots in the top ends of the splint.

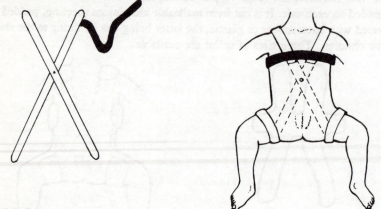

Fig. 7.6 Barlow splint.

The Barlow splint is applied in a similar way to that described for the von Rosen splint. The upper ends are moulded over the shoulders where they are held together with the canvas strap which passes around the child's chest (Fig. 7.6). The lower ends of the splint are moulded around the thighs after reduction of the hip, with the hips in a position of 90 degrees of flexion, and not more than 45 degrees of abduction.

One complication of the Barlow splint is that as the two aluminium strips are joined by only a single rivet, the upper ends of the splint may press against the sides of the child's neck as the child moves.

MANAGEMENT OF A CHILD IN A VON ROSEN OR BARLOW SPLINT

— Instruct the mother not to take the child out of the splint. The child is tended and washed in the splint.
— Examine the child at weekly intervals, adjusting the splint as necessary.

- Replace the splint with a larger one when necessary. When a larger splint is being applied the hips must be kept in abduction, flexion and lateral rotation. This can be accomplished by lying the child on its abdomen while the splint is being changed.
- Discard the splint after twelve weeks and take a radiograph.
- Examine the child at weekly intervals for the first six weeks after discarding the splint, then at decreasing intervals until six months have elapsed.
- Take a radiograph of the child's hips when he is six months old. If the radiograph is normal, see the child at one-yearly intervals. If the radiograph shows a difference in the acetabular angle on the affected side, take further radiographs at yearly intervals until normal development of the acetabulum has occurred.

FREJKA PILLOW (Frejka, 1954)

The Frejka pillow (Fig. 7.7) consists of a firm rectangular pad filled with feathers or kapok which may be divided transversely into three sections. Attached to the upper end of the pad are two long straps, joined in the region of the scapulae, which pass over the shoulders to be reattached by buckles to the lower end of the pad. There are two shorter straps which pass around the sides of the trunk.

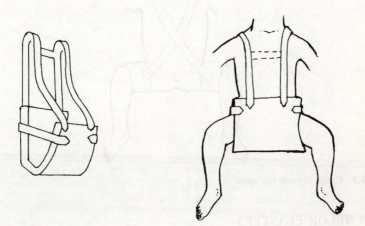

Fig. 7.7 Frejka pillow.

Frejka originally introduced this appliance in 1938, and since 1946 has used it regularly as the method of choice in the treatment of children in the first year of life. He claims that the dislocated femoral head slips spontaneously and without any manipulation into the acetabulum. The disadvantage of the Frejka pillow is that it can cause damage to the capital femoral epiphysis (Ilfeld and Makin, 1977) and it must be removed frequently to clean and bathe the child.

DENIS BROWNE HIP SPLINT (Browne, 1948)

In this splint (Figs 7.8, 7.9) the child's hips are held in abduction/flexion and lateral rotation, the range of movement possible in each direction being about 30 degrees. The splint does not have to be removed to keep the child clean. Crawling and later walking are possible in this splint. One important advantage of the splint as opposed to immobilisation in a plaster cast, is that it will not retain an unstable reduction as the hip redislocates, thus enabling the surgeon to recognise this condition early rather than late (Lloyd Roberts, 1971).

After the splint is removed, the legs slowly adduct to the neutral position during the subsequent four to six weeks.

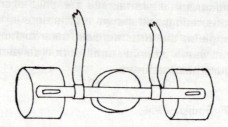

Fig. 7.8 Denis Browne hip splint seen from behind.

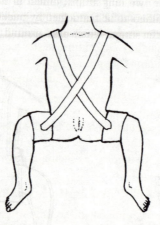

Fig. 7.9 Denis Browne hip splint.

BATCHELOR PLASTERS

Batchelor plasters hold the hips in abduction and medial rotation. They encircle the lower limbs only and extend from the groins to the ankles being joined by a crossbar (Fig. 7.10). The knees must be held in 15 to 20 degrees of flexion to prevent rotation of the limbs within the plaster casts.

A possible complication of the use of Batchelor plasters is an increase in the degree of anteversion of the femoral necks (Wilkinson, 1963), which may have to be corrected subsequently by derotation osteotomies of the upper ends of the femora.

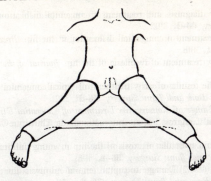

Fig. 7.10 Batchelor plasters.

FROG OR LORENZ PLASTER CAST

This cast (Fig. 7.11) was originally described as holding the hips in a position of 90 degrees of abduction/flexion and lateral rotation. The immobilisation of a hip in this position has been shown to increase the risk of the development of avascular necrosis of the femoral capital epiphysis (Allen, 1962; Gore, 1974), and therefore this position must not be used. The hips can be flexed to 90 degrees but must not be abducted beyond 45 degrees. It must be possible to place the hips easily in the desired position before applying the cast. If the adductor muscles are tight, a subcutaneous tenotomy at their origin must be carried out.

Unlike the von Rosen and Barlow splints, the cast is not generally used in the management of the dislocated hip in the newborn. The cast extends from the nipple line down to the ankles on both sides, leaving the ankles and feet free. Particular care must be taken to ensure that the cast is strong enough over the groins and buttocks. If it is not, the cast easily cracks due to the stresses imposed upon it by the strong movements of the child's limbs. An adequate opening must be allowed around the perineum to enable the child to be kept clean.

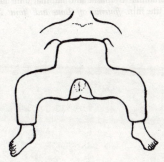

Fig. 7.11 Frog or Lorenz plaster cast.

REFERENCES

Allen, R.P. (1962) Ischaemicnecrosis following treatment of hip dysplasia. *Journal of the American Medical Association,* **180,** 497.
Andren, L. & Rosen, S. von (1958) The diagnosis of dislocation of the hip in newborns and the primary results of immediate treatment. *Acta Radiologica,* **49,** 89.

Barlow, T.G. (1962) Early diagnosis and treatment of congenital dislocation of hip. *Journal of Bone and Joint Surgery*, **44-B,** 292.

Browne, D. (1948) The treatment of congenital dislocation of the hip. *Proceedings of the Royal Society of Medicine*, **41,** 388.

Erlacher, P.J. (1962) Early treatment of dysplasia of the hip. *Journal of the International College of Surgeons*, **38,** 348.

Fredensborg, N. (1976) The results of early treatment of typical congenital dislocation of the hip in Malmö. *Journal of Bone and Joint Surgery*, **58-B,** 272.

Frejka, M.B. (1954) *The Danger of Conservative Treatment of Congenital Dislocation of the Hip*. p. 573. Sixth International Congress Societe Internationale de Chirurgie Orthopedique et de Traumatologie.

Gore, D.R. (1974) Iatrogenic avascular necrosis of the hip in young children: a review of six cases. *Journal of Bone and Joint Surgery*, **56-A,** 493.

Ilfeld, F.W. & Makin, M. (1977) Damage to capital femoral epiphysis due to Frejka pillow treatment. *Journal of Bone and Joint Surgery*, **59-A,** 654.

Lloyd-Roberts, G.C. (1971) *Orthopaedics in Infancy and Childhood*, p. 218. London: Butterworth.

Nelson, M.A. (1966) Early diagnosis of congenital dislocation of the hip. *Journal of Bone and Joint Surgery*, **48-B,** 388.

Nicholson, J.T., Kopell, H.P. & Mattei, F.A. (1954) Regional stress angiography of the hip: A preliminary report. *Journal of Bone and Joint Surgery*, **36-A,** 503.

Ogden, J.A. & Southwick, W.O. (1973) A possible cause of avascular necrosis complicating the treatment of congenital dislocation of the hip. *Journal of Bone and Joint Surgery*, **55-A,** 1770.

Ogden, J.A. (1974) Patterns of proximal femoral vascularity. *Journal of Bone and Joint Surgery*, **56-A,** 941.

Ortolani, M. (1948) *La Lussazione Congenita Dell'anca. Nuovi Criteri Diagnostici e Profilattico-Correttivi*, p. 19, figs 1–4; p. 20, figs 5, 6; p. 21, fig. 7. Bologna: Cappelli.

Ramsey, P. L., Lasser, S. & MacEwen, G.D. (1976) Congenital dislocation of the hip. Use of Pavlik harness in the child during the first six months of life. *Journal of Bone and Joint Surgery*, **58-A,** 1000.

Rosen, S. von (1956) Early diagnosis and treatment of congenital dislocation of the hip joint. *Acta Orthopaedica Scandinavica*, **26,** 136.

Rosen, S. von (1962) Diagnosis and treatment of congenital dislocation of the hip joint in the new-born. *Journal of Bone and Joint Surgery*, **44-B,** 284.

Salter, R.B. & Field, P. (1960) The effects of continuous compression on living articular cartilage. *Journal of Bone and Joint Surgery*, **42-A,** 31.

Westin, G.W., Ilfeld, F.W. & Provost, J. (1976) Total avascular necrosis of the capital femoral epiphysis in congenital dislocated hips. *Clinical Orthopaedics and Related Research*, **119,** 93.

Wilkinson, J.A. (1963) Prime factors in the aetiology of congenital dislocation of the hip. *Journal of Bone and Joint Surgery*, **45-B,** 268.

Wynne-Davies, R. (1970) Acetabular dysplasia and familial joint laxity: two aetiological factors in congenital dislocation of the hip. *Journal of Bone and Joint Surgery*, **52-B,** 704.

8.

Management of patients in traction

Patients in traction and traction-suspension systems do not look after themselves.
The correct management of patients in traction depends upon team work if good results are to be obtained. Sustained interest and effort is required from every member of the team — medical, nursing, physiotherapy and other paramedical staff — looking after the patient. No one aspect of patient care is the sole responsibility of an individual member of the team although certain procedures will normally be carried out by one member of the team because of training and expertise. All members of the team must be aware of potential problems and complications, and must see that any that do develop are dealt with immediately, either by themselves or by another, more expert, member of the team. Thus adjustments to the traction-suspension system may be made by the nursing staff at the suggestion of the doctors, and medical complications may be brought to the attention of the doctors by other members of the team.

A member of the medical staff must examine the patient and the traction-suspension system every morning and evening. The nursing staff, who are in constant attendance, must observe closely both the patient and the traction-suspension system, as their intimate knowledge of the patient can enable them to detect minor changes in the patient's appearance and demeanour, which may herald the development of complications. A physiotherapist must visit daily, both to treat the patient and to ensure that the patient carries out a sensible regime of exercises on his own. Occupational therapists, teachers, dieticians, social workers and the rehabilitation officer will be asked to visit when appropriate.

Daily checks must be made to ensure that the patient is comfortable, that complications are not occurring, and that the traction-suspension system is achieving the desired effect. The patient, and the traction-suspension system must be examined. Regular radiological examinations of the position of the fracture must be made. The radiographs must be inspected and action taken if the position is not satisfactory. Physiotherapy to the whole patient, as well as to the injured part, is vital to ensure that when the fracture has united, the general condition of the patient, as well as the condition of the injured limb are such that full function is regained as quickly as possible.

Lastly, at some stage, the decision must be taken whether to discard traction completely and mobilise the patient, or to change to another method of treatment.

THE PATIENT

NURSING CARE

Patients on traction need all the usual care given to every patient in hospital. In addition, extra attention must be paid to certain areas.

General appearance
The nursing staff have the best opportunity to observe the patient. Careful note must be taken of changes in manner and appearance, which may not be apparent to other staff. A fine petechial rash and unexpected confusion or aggression, for example, may indicate the onset of fat embolism. It must be remembered that long term orthopaedic patients can develop non-orthopaedic conditions such as influenza or appendicitis.

Observations and charts
In the early stages after a fracture, a careful record must be kept of the patient's temperature, pulse, respiration and blood pressure, as these may indicate the necessity for blood transfusion, antibiotic or other therapy. In the later stages of treatment, daily recording of observations should be sufficient.

Bed and bedding
The bed must be of adequate length for the patient and of convenient height for the nursing staff. It must have a rigid base for the mattress or a fracture board between the mattress and the springs. It must provide a firm base for the attachment of the Balkan beam or pulleys.

If possible, plastic draw sheets should be avoided, to reduce sweating and skin maceration. Creases and crumbs are uncomfortable and predispose to bed sores. Bed cradles are needed to prevent bedding pressing down on toes. When one leg is in traction, bedding must be arranged to cover the sound leg whilst leaving the injured leg unencumbered for traction and exercises. This will be the case also when a split bed frame and mattress are used in Perkins traction (see p. 28). Bed socks are often needed on the exposed foot. Back rests must work and be secure. Several pillows are often required. When the patient wishes to sleep, the backrest and pillows may need to be adjusted so that the patient can lie down. The nursing staff must check that there is sufficient freedom of movement in the traction-suspension system to allow the patient to change position, and instruct the patient how to do so without upsetting the system.

A 'monkey pole' is essential. It is a short bar which hangs above the patient where it can be grabbed easily so that he can lift his trunk off the bed. It must be strong enough to support the whole weight of the patient. The bar may be slung from a hook in the ceiling, from a gantry at the head end of the bed or from a Balkan beam.

Food

A balanced mixed diet is needed, with the usual proportions of protein, fat, carbohydrate, vitamins and minerals. There does not seem to be any virtue in special additions to the diet. As some patients will be in hospital for a long time, it is easy for the diet to become monotonous. Care must be taken to avoid this. Overeating must be avoided, as an increase in weight may make subsequent mobilisation more difficult. Occasionally a weight-reducing diet will be required.

The mechanics of eating may require some thought, especially if the patient cannot sit up. Flexible straws, bowls and one-handed eating utensils can help. Water jugs must be placed within reach on properly positioned bed tables or lockers. When both arms are injured, the patient may have to be fed initially.

Toilet

All toilet functions have to be performed in bed. Adequate facilities and privacy must be provided — urinals, slipper bedpans, splash receivers, and extra screens where bulky traction apparatus will not allow the normal curtains to close around the bed. The traction-suspension system must enable the patient to get on and off a bedpan with the minimum of pain and effort. Catheterisation may be necessary to avoid bed sores which can result from urinary incontinence.

Pain relief

Fractures can be very painful in the early stages. It is therefore very important that adequate analgesia is prescribed *and given*. Where essential nursing and physiotherapy procedures cause unavoidable pain, extra analgesia is required. Injections should be replaced by oral medication as soon as practicable. Long term opiates must be avoided.

Skin

Bed sores are a potential complication of prolonged bed rest. This may be a greater problem in patients in traction because these patients initially are unable or reluctant to move. In severely injured patients, regular turning or lifting must begin soon after admission. The traction-suspension system itself can cause local pressure problems. Skin must be kept clean and dry, and be inspected regularly wherever pressure could cause problems. Synthetic sheepskin, foam plastic leg troughs and heel pads can help. The provision of these aids is only a part of proper nursing care and not a substitute for the personal attention that is still required.

Mental state

Patients in traction are frequently anxious. It is important to try to minimize this, by explaining the aims of their treatment, the function of the various items of equipment and the reason for carrying out exercises. An estimate of the expected duration of treatment should be given with a warning that a longer period of treatment will be required if initial healing is delayed. This will enable the patient to plan his work and family life, and help prevent the serious depression that can result from being told that several more weeks in traction are needed when the expectation had been that treatment was complete. Patients may need professional help to sort out the financial and legal consequences of their accident. At a fairly early stage they may ask for an estimate of the severity of their final disability and any likely deformity. They may be unpleasantly surprised to hear that they have damaged themselves permanently, and may welcome the opportunity to discuss this realistically.

Many patients in traction are young and fit apart from their injury, which soon becomes painless. They must be kept alert and occupied to prevent boredom. It is important that the hospital radio equipment works and is within reach, and that personal radio and television sets have earphones to avoid inconvenience to other patients. Arrangements must be made for bookrests and page holders if the patient is in an unusual position; mirrors if the patient has to lie flat, prone, or keep his neck stiff, so that he can see what is going on around him and who is approaching him; bed tables for handicrafts or modelmaking; a 'long arm' to pick up things dropped on the floor; patients with similar interests to be beside one another; children and students to continue their education with arrangements for work to be brought in by tutors and teachers, regular hours being set aside for this; adults, who will be unable to return to their previous occupation, to start their retraining by studying while in bed.

Communication

The nursing staff often will have to explain again what the doctors have told the patients about their treatment. They may be asked the same questions. It is important that all members of the team have discussed the problem so that they will all give substantially the same answers. Patients will often mention to the nursing staff, worries that they are reluctant to discuss directly with the medical staff, but be grateful when they are discussed.

Relatives often will need explanations and reassurance when they see traction apparatus. People confined to hospital for a long time need the support and interest of their visitors. Visiting must be made easy, but restricted if the patient tires easily. At all times a friendly watch must be kept to prevent children or playful adults jolting the patient, swinging the traction weights or decorating the cords in such a way as to interfere with their function.

MEDICAL CARE

Blood loss

Broken bones bleed. The bleeding usually is concealed within the limb or trunk, with the result that it is easy to underestimate the volume of blood which has been lost.

The following table gives the minimum amounts that are likely to have been lost in 'average' closed fractures. It also gives the range of values for fractures of different severity.

Table 8.1

Closed shaft fractures	Range of blood lost	Minimum average loss
Tibia	500–1000 ml	500 ml (1 pint)
Femur — shaft	1500–2500 ml	1500 ml (3 pints)
Pelvis	2000–exsanguination	2000 ml (4 pints)
Humerus	500–1000 ml	500 ml (1 pint)

If the fracture is badly comminuted or compound, at least an extra 500 ml is added to the above amounts. These figures are based on the work of Clarke et al (1961) at the Birmingham Accident Hospital.

If several bones are fractured the separate estimated losses are added together to calculate the total volume of blood to be transfused. In severe cases this may exceed the normal circulating blood volume.

When it is anticipated that a large volume of blood will be needed a filter should be used to lessen the risk of post traumatic respiratory insufficiency — or shock lung. It is thought that dead cells and debris from stored blood may contribute to congestion in the lungs. The condition is described with further references in Rockwood and Green (1975).

In most fractures 50% of the total blood loss occurs in the first 2 to 5 hours after injury (Clark et al, 1961), but femoral fractures bleed for longer. With all fractures further transfusion may be required if haemoglobin estimations show the late development of anaemia.

Overtransfusion with consequent cardiac failure can occur when the volume of blood lost has been overestimated, or replacement infusions have been given too quickly. The elderly are most at risk.

Chest complications

A supine or semi-recumbent position will predispose to poor ventilation of the lungs, sputum retention, lobar collapse and infection, especially in the elderly.

Sudden collapse with breathlessness and cyanosis may be the result of a massive pulmonary embolism from venous thrombosis. Smaller or recurrent emboli may be present with gradual deterioration in mental function, fevers, pleuritic chest pain and cough. Chest radiographs, estimation of the blood gases and a lung scan may support a clinical diagnosis.

A fat embolism usually occurs soon after the original injury or a major adjustment of the position of the fracture. One of the earliest signs may be a change in the behaviour or mental state of the patient. This presentation can be confused easily with the effects of alcohol withdrawal in heavy drinkers, the latter tends to occur after the same time interval. Fat embolism is sometimes accompanied by a petechial rash over the upper trunk, but this may be transient and therefore easily missed. An estimation of the blood gases is one of the most useful diagnostic tests — the partial pressure of oxygen may be dramatically lowered — although this will not differentiate it from a pulmonary embolism.

Urinary tract

Incomplete emptying of the bladder, due to the unaccustomed position predisposes to urinary infection. Incontinence may result in the elderly and prove a distressing and troublesome complication.

Acute renal failure can occur as a result of inadequate restoration of the circulating blood volume. Urinary output in the days following a major injury must be measured.

The recumbent position leads to urinary stasis with the result that calculi can form in the kidneys and bladder. Traction must be arranged so that the patient can easily alter his position. Beds should be tipped if possible. A good fluid intake and urinary output is encouraged.

Bowels

Constipation is likely due to inactivity, the difficulty of using bed pans and perhaps the effect of opiate analgesia. If allowed to persist, it can lead to faecal impaction and spurious diarrhoea as well as large bowel obstruction.

Pre-existing conditions

Pregnancy may add an extra dimension to the management of some patients. Treatment may have to be modified as a result. The insulin requirements of a patient with diabetes mellitus may be altered.

Patients with pathological fractures due to metabolic bone disease or large doses of steroid may present special problems. If a patient's normal dosage of vitamin D is continued, hypercalcaemia can occur. Steroids cannot be stopped in most cases. They often however contribute to delay in bone and soft tissue healing.

CARE OF THE INJURED LIMB

The injured limb must be examined twice daily. Where there is pain, soreness, discharge or odour, bandages, must be removed or a window cut in a plaster cast to enable close examination of the underlying limb. It is better to lose the position of the fracture than to ignore the possible development of a serious complication.

Pain

This may result from pressure sores developing in the groin, around the ankle, under the strapping or over the sacrum, or infection of a pin track or a compound fracture. In children, who are being managed in modified Bryant's traction for congenital dislocation of the hip, pain may result from impingement of the femoral head on the superior lip of the acetabulum.

Paraesthesia or numbness

This may result from impairment of normal nerve function by ischaemia, pressure or excessive traction on a nerve.

Skin irritation

This comes from allergy to adhesive strapping.

Swelling

This may be caused by the development of deep vein thrombosis, lack of exercise or a bandage being applied too tightly.

Weakness of ankle, toe, wrist or finger movement

This may result from impairment of nerve function, disuse and muscular atrophy. The ulnar nerve at the elbow and the common peroneal nerve at the neck of the fibula are particularly at risk.

Reduced range of dorsiflexion of the ankle joint
This comes from contraction of the calf muscles and the posterior capsule of the joint, and may occur if the foot is allowed to lie in plantarflexion.

Painful limitation of dorsiflexion of the hallux
This suggests ischaemia of the flexor hallucis longus muscle; that of the fingers, ischaemia of the deep flexor muscles of the forearm. It must be remembered that the circulation in muscles can be impaired even although the peripheral pulses are palpable.

Much can be deduced about the condition of the fracture by clinical examination. Inspection, palpation and the careful use of a tape measure will usually show the presence of overlap, angulation or mal-rotation at the fracture site. Mal-rotation is detected more easily by clinical than radiological examination. In the lower limb, the anterior superior iliac spine, the middle of the patella and the first interdigital cleft are usually in a straight line. This can be checked on the un-injured limb. If the limb is obviously short there must be overlap or angulation at the fracture site or dislocation of a neighbouring joint.

The resolution of the haematoma at the fracture site and its conversion into callus can be followed by palpation. Pain at rest and on movement at the fracture site passes off within a few days. As healing progresses towards union, the fracture site becomes less tender and movements decrease and ultimately disappear. In the early stages clinical examination is a better guide to progress than radiographic examination.

THE TRACTION SUSPENSION SYSTEM

The traction-suspension-system must be checked DAILY, and after each period of physiotherapy or radiographic examination.

Bed and Balkan beam
Regular checks are needed to ensure that the Balkan beam is firmly fixed to the bed and that all clamps and brackets are secure. If a spanner is required for this, it must always be hanging on the bed.

If sliding traction is used the bed must be elevated at one end or side so that the pull of the traction weights is opposed by gravity acting on the patient's weight. If elevation is not provided, the patient will be dragged in the direction of the traction weights, causing discomfort and skin friction. For skull traction the head of the bed is elevated. For most other forms of sliding traction, the foot of the bed is elevated. If the bed cannot be tipped, bed blocks or some other form of elevating frame must be provided.

Splints
The position of the ring of a Thomas's or similar splint must be checked as it can slip down the thigh. If the splint is continually slipping down the thigh, the suspension cords must be adjusted to give an increased pull directed towards the

head of the bed. The skin under the ring of a splint must be examined as it, or injudiciously placed cords, may rub in the groin. The ring of a splint often becomes loose when the swelling associated with the fracture settles. If the ring is not adjustable, the splint may have to be changed to one with a smaller ring. Only the ring of a Thomas's splint should rest on the bed.

The limb must be kept away from the side bars of the splint — a common peroneal nerve palsy can easily occur. Any clamps on the splint must be tight and hinges must move freely.

Slings and padding

Even the most skillfully placed slings and padding become wrinkled and displaced after a few days. It may be necessary to remove the bandages supporting the limb on the splint to allow the underlying limb to be examined. After the first few days, little discomfort will be caused to the patient by minor movements at the fracture site, so that it is easy to reposition padding. Slings can be tightened or loosened readily as long as the plan of attachment detailed on page 14 has been followed. The safety pins or toothed clips are removed and the cloth slings tightened or loosened until the position of the fracture and limb looks and feels correct; the pins or clips are then replaced. Any padding which has become wet, soiled or lumpy is changed. The back of the heel and the tendo calcaneus are inspected for evidence of pressure sores. The most distal sling under the leg, must lie at least $2\frac{1}{2}$ inches (6.0 cm) above the insertion of the tendo calcaneus.

Skin traction

If adhesive skin traction is being used, it must not be wrinkled, cause an allergic skin reaction or slide down the limb as a result of excessive traction being applied to it.

If non-adhesive skin traction is used, it may need to be re-applied frequently, as it may slip down the limb.

The encircling bandage must be firmly applied, but must not embarrass the circulation. The malleoli must be checked for pressure or evidence of friction from the skin traction. The spreader bar to which the traction cords are attached should lie 4–6 inches (10–15 cm) beyond the ankle or wrist to allow freedom of movement of the foot or hand.

If the skin becomes sore, skin traction must be discontinued.

Skeletal traction

Skeletal traction should not be painful. The pins or wire used for the application of skeletal traction must be immobile in the bone. The skin wounds must be dry and not inflamed. If the skin wounds are moist or inflamed, or the pin is loose in the bone, infection of the pin track may be present or imminent. When a pin track is infected, percussion over the bone through which the pin or wire passes, is painful.

When infection of the pin track is present, the pin must be removed as soon as possible. A decision must then be taken either to replace the pin with another at a different site, to substitute skin traction, or to discontinue traction completely.

Generally it is not advisable to try to persevere with skeletal traction in the presence of infection even with antibiotic cover.

The type of pin in use must be recorded so that the correct technique can be used in its removal. A Steinmann pin can be pulled out easily and painlessly without analgesia using a chuck handle to grip the blunt end, after the sharp end has been cleaned thoroughly. A Denham pin has to be unscrewed until the threaded portion is clear of the bone and skin. This can be painful if suitable analgesia is not given.

Stirrups

The Böhler stirrup used to attach a traction cord to a Steinmann or Denham pin must be clamped securely to the pin so that it does not slip sideways and press on the skin, causing skin necrosis and infection. This is more likely to occur if the pin has been inserted obliquely to the long axis of the limb. The stirrup must rotate freely on its swivels. These often require lubrication. Because of the proximity of the skin wounds, it is best to use either sterilized petroleum jelly or liquid paraffin. The pin must not rotate with the stirrup, otherwise the pin will become loose and infection of the pin track occur.

The Kirschner wire strainer clamps firmly to the Kirschner wire, and therefore movement of the strainer is imparted to the wire. To ensure that the strainer does not become detached from the wire, strapping can be applied around the locking lugs.

The arch of the stirrup must not be allowed to rest on the limb otherwise pressure necrosis of the underlying skin will occur. The shin is the site most at risk.

Cords

The colour coding of cords performing different functions has been suggested (see p. 57) — red or green for traction cords and white for suspension cords. The cords must be attached firmly by standard knots which can be seen easily. The point of attachment of the cords must not have moved and all knots must be secure. Knots should be avoided in the length of any cord, to prevent it jamming in a pulley. If a cord is too short, it is better to replace it completely. If it is too long it can be shortened at the weight end. All cords, traction and suspension, must be of adequate length to allow the patient freedom of movement. To prevent fraying, the ends of the cords can be bound with adhesive tape or heat sealed if they are of nylon. Cords can also fray where they move over pulleys or if they are allowed to rub against each other. This is more likely with vigorous physiotherapy. The line of pull of the cords must be checked to ensure that the correct pull is being applied to the fracture, and that any splint is kept in its correct position.

Pulleys

Pulleys must be of as large a diameter as possible to reduce friction and be free running. Some may require occasional lubrication. They must be attached firmly to the Balkan beam. The cords must rest comfortably in the pulleys to minimise friction and fraying.

If a multiple pulley system is used, the mechanical advantage of the system must be known, so that the correct weight is applied. In the example shown in Figure 4.3, a weight of 5 lb (2.3 kg) exerts a pull of 10 lb (4.6 kg) at C.

Weights

These come in many forms from cloth bags filled with sand, to metal weights and hangers. The weight used must be known and must include the weight of any hanger. They must hang free and not rest on the floor or catch on the bed when the patient moves. It is sometimes necessary to hang weights over the patient. These must always have an extra safety cord, separate from the traction-suspension system, so that the weight cannot fall onto the patient. Weights which have to be removed to facilitate physiotherapy should be held by clips so that they are easily removable.

RADIOGRAPHIC EXAMINATION

When a fracture is managed in either fixed or sliding traction, regular radiographic examination with two exposures taken at right angles to each other is essential throughout the period of immobilisation, to ensure that reduction of the fracture is achieved and maintained until union occurs. It is important that the traction-suspension system is arranged in such a way that the radiographer is able to position her machine close enough to the patient to take the views requested. She must be told which parts of the system can be moved and which parts must be left undisturbed. If the patient is to go to the radiology department, instructions must be given as to whether the traction is to be left in place or removed during transit and radiography. A rough guide to the frequency of radiographic examination is:

> Two or three times in the first week while adjustments are
>   being made to the traction, then
> Weekly for the next three weeks, then
> Monthly until union occurs
> After each manipulation of the fracture
> After each change in the traction weight.

PHYSIOTHERAPY

Hugh Owen Thomas (1876) emphasised the 'combination of enforced, uninterrupted and prolonged rest; the first gives relief from pain, the second, added to the first, enables the case steadily to progress to a cure, and the third secures that which has been gained' whereas Lucas-Championnière (1895) believed that the full function of a limb returned earlier if muscle and joint contractures were prevented. This latter view is fully supported by Perkins (1970). The correct management of a fracture depends upon obtaining a balance between these two concepts so that the fracture unites in the best functional position as rapidly as possible, the development of joint stiffness is prevented or minimised, as much muscle power as possible is retained, demineralisation of the skeleton is minimal, and the risk of pneumonia, venous thrombosis and renal calculi is decreased (British Orthopaedic Association, 1955).

The mental and physical condition of the whole patient as well as the condition of the injured limb is very important. Rehabilitation is begun immediately, its intensity increasing as union of the fracture progresses, becoming maximal when union has occurred.

The traction-suspension system employed in the management of a fracture should allow as much activity of the patient as possible, consistent with the requirements of the fracture itself. Every patient must be encouraged repeatedly to be as active as possible. Many patients being treated in traction-suspension systems are afraid that they will upset the system or the reduction of the fracture if they move. It must be emphasised that this will not occur. If it does, the fault is that of the doctor who set up the system, and not that of the patient.

The physiotherapist is an important member of the team, and must have full information about the patient. This information is obtained from the patient's notes and X-rays, the ward sister and her nursing records, and personal contact with the doctors in charge of the patient. It is not sufficient to rely upon written request forms. Having been told the diagnosis, the aims of treatment and whether the traction weights can be reduced or removed temporarily, the physiotherapist will devise the best programme of treatment for the patient in consultation with her senior colleagues and the other members of the team. In addition because of her close daily contact with the patient she is well placed to observe and report upon the early development of any complications which may need medical treatment, such as chest infection, deep vein thrombosis or those affecting the fracture.

Emphasis is placed upon coughing and breathing exercises to keep the lungs clear and to encourage venous return from the limbs. Ankle and leg exercises will help to prevent deep vein thrombosis. Bad posture in bed, which could lead to backache, must be avoided. Part of each day should be spent lying flat to avoid the development of hip contractures. Joint stiffness and progressive weakening from disuse must be prevented by a programme of exercises. Once taught these can be done by the patient without supervision. If sufficient patients with similar problems can be grouped together in the ward, an element of competition can be introduced as an incentive. Any apparatus, such as weights and springs, which may be needed must be available for use at all times.

Initially treatment of the injured limb is directed to the reduction of swelling in preparation for subsequent movement. As soon as possible the patient must be encouraged to contract the muscles affected by the fracture or joint injury. Isometric contraction can be used if movement causes pain. Quadriceps exercises are important for injuries around the knee. They must be felt to contract. Exercises for the hamstring muscles must be carried out also.

After removal of the traction, all patients should have a period of time free in bed, during which they can develop confidence in their injured limb. The method of ambulation to be employed must be explained to them, and they must be warned that initially they could tire easily.

Patients often complain of pain in their feet when they first walk after a long period of time in bed. A board in the bed against which they can press their feet may help to prevent this.

It must be possible to transport easily to the ward, all the equipment to be used by the physiotherapist. Sandbags which may be used to steady the limb in the early stages when parts of the traction are removed, can also be used along with weight boots and springs, by the patient to do his own exercises.

Slippery boards are a great help in knee flexion exercises, when a split bed frame is not in use, as the heel of the injured leg slides more easily on the board than on the bed clothes.

Ice should always be readily available, as it is very helpful in relieving pain and reducing swellings and effusions. It should be used for short periods and the skin protected with medical paraffin oil. The ice must always be wet and wrapped in a wet towel. This aids heat exchange and prevents the temperature dropping below freezing, with the attendant risk of ice burns. Ice must not be used if skin sensation is abnormal.

Ultrasound will help haematomata, which are not at the fracture site, to disperse.

REMOVAL OF TRACTION

The decision when to remove traction, is a compromise between the earliest possible ambulation and the avoidance of complications at the fracture site such as angulation, shortening and refracture.

It is now common practice to continue traction until the fracture is stable, and then to change to another method of supporting the fracture until union has occurred. A fracture is stable when any deformity which is produced at the fracture site by a deforming force, tends to disappear when that force is removed. Thus in many stable fractures, movement at the fracture site, including telescoping on axial compression, can be present. If movement causes pain or the deformity does not disappear on removal of the deforming force, the fracture is not stable, and permanent deformity may result if traction is discontinued at this stage.

If it is not proposed to substitute another method of supporting the fracture when traction is removed, then traction will have to be continued for a longer period of time. Shortening, angulation and refracture are likely to occur if there is definite tenderness of the callus or movement at the fracture site; radiographs show that only a small amount of callus is present, or is located mainly on one side of the fracture, or fine cracks are present in the cortex of one or other of the major fragments (Seimon, 1964). Charnley (1970) states that the occurrence of late angulation or spontaneous refracture of the femur is preceded by a decrease in the range of knee flexion. He suggests that there should be an initial period when the range of knee flexion is measured daily.

The following are examples of the length of time which adults might require to spend in traction for different fractures:

Elbow fracture with olecranon pin	3 weeks
Tibial fracture with calcaneal pin	3–6 weeks
(if traction is removed at 3 weeks it may be	
advisable to incorporate the pin in a long	
leg plaster cast, and then remove it at 6	
weeks when a new cast is applied)	
Trochanteric fracture of the femur, allowing	
partial weight-bearing	6 weeks
Femoral shaft fracture	
with application of cast brace and partial	
weight-bearing	6 weeks
without external support and partial	
weight-bearing	12 weeks

REFERENCES

British Orthopaedic Association (1955) Debate on 'That Lucas-Championnière was right', British Orthopaedic Association Meeting, Liverpool, October 7, 1955. *Journal of Bone and Joint Surgery,* **37-B,** 719.

Charnley, J. (1970) *The Closed Treatment of Common Fractures,* p. 189, 3rd edn. Edinburgh: Churchill Livingstone.

Clarke, R., Fisher, M.R., Topley, E. & Davies, J.W.L. (1961) Extent and time of blood loss after civilian injury. *Lancet,* **ii,** 381.

Lucas-Championnière, J. (1895) *Traitement des Fractures par le Massage et la Mobilisation.* Paris: Rueff.

Perkins, G. (1970) *The Ruminations of an Orthopaedic Surgeon.* London: Butterworth.

Rockwood, C.A. & Green, D.P. (1975) Post Traumatic Respiratory Insufficiency, p. 159. In *Fractures.* Philadelphia: Lippincott.

Seimon, L.P. (1964) Refracture of the shaft of the femur. *Journal of Bone and Joint Surgery,* **46-B,** 32.

Thomas, H.O. (1876) *Diseases of the Hip, Knee and Ankle Joints, with their Deformities, Treated by a New and Efficient Method,* p. iii, 2nd edn. Liverpool: Dobb.

9.

Prescription of orthoses

The term orthotics encompasses the provision of splints and appliances which improve the function and appearance of a patient. An orthosis is an appliance which is added to the patient, to enable better use to be made of that part of the body to which it is fitted, whereas a prosthesis replaces a missing part of the body.

An orthosis is prescribed by a doctor with a specific aim in mind. With regard to the lower limbs, the main functions of which are to support the trunk and propulsion, the aim of prescribing an orthosis is to improve these functions by providing stability, overcoming weakness, relieving pain and controlling deformities. To achieve this an orthosis must be as strong, light, simple and easy to apply and manipulate as possible. In addition it should be cosmetically acceptable to the patient. Occasionally operations are necessary to correct deformities, in order to simplify the manufacture and fitting of an orthosis. The prescription therefore must state clearly the disability for which the orthosis is to compensate, or the deformity which it is to correct; the anatomical limits of the orthosis; and the direction and type of forces which the orthosis is to exert.

The orthotist receives the prescription, measures the patient, designs the most suitable form of the prescribed orthosis and then makes out a detailed order specifying the materials, exact measurements and details of fitting. He may take a plaster cast of the patient's limb or trunk to enable an exact model to be made, upon which the orthosis can be constructed.

The detailed order form from the orthotist is sent to a workshop where the manufacturer's technician has to rely completely upon the information supplied by the orthotist, as he may never see the patient and may be in another part of the country altogether. This arrangement can cause difficulties, delays and frustrations. The ideal solution is when the orthotist discusses the problem with the doctor, sees the patient, takes his own measurements and constructs and fits the appliance himself.

When the orthosis is completed and finally fitted, the prescribing doctor must check that the orthosis complies with his original wishes, and does in fact help the patient. Only then is payment to the manufacturer authorised by the doctor's signature.

The doctor and the orthotist must work closely together. Frequent discussions are needed to clarify all but the most meticulous prescription if the patient is to receive most benefit, and unnecessary cost is to be avoided. Personal contact is always better than complicated forms, as a means of communication.

DEVELOPMENT OF ORTHOTIC TERMINOLOGY

There has been a recent revolution in the approved terminology for orthoses. This has been accepted in some areas and has met with firm resistance in others.

There have always been many different types of splints and appliances with even more modifications, because of patients' varying size, shape and disability. To avoid lengthy descriptions of appliances, the name of the inventor or his institution was often used for brevity. The name did not necessarily describe the function of the splint or even its site on the body. Over the years, the named appliances frequently were modified until it became impossible to be certain in which form the appliance would be supplied when ordered by name. Sometimes this resulted in unsatisfactory orthoses being supplied. In addition it was not possible to work out a standard schedule of fees for use in North America.

Committees, from interested bodies in the United States of America, were established to try to introduce a more logical method of prescribing orthoses. Although knowledge and understanding of the underlying pathological process affecting the musculo-skeletal system is important in the prognosis and overall care of the patient, differing pathological processes can result in the same biomechanical defects. Technical analysis forms were developed. On these forms the patient's sensory, motor and skeletal defects are detailed graphically. This enables an orthosis to be prescribed on the basis of the patient's functional disability and the objectives of the treatment.

TECHNICAL ANALYSIS FORMS

There are four different technical analysis forms, one for the lower limbs (Fig. 9.1), one for the spine and one each for the left and right upper limb (see Appendix 2), all of a size which can be accommodated easily in a patient's notes.

Each form consists of four pages. On the first page, details of the patient are entered. These include his name, age and unit number as well as his ambulatory status and any major skeletal, sensory, motor or vascular impairment. At the bottom of the first page there is a legend of symbols which are used when completing the second and third pages of the form.

On the second and third pages, there are skeletal outlines of the spine, lower limbs and upper limb depending upon the form. Circles, divided into 30 degree segments, are drawn over the major joints in the upper and lower limbs. Shaded areas represent the normal ranges of movement present at these joints. In the lower limb form (Fig. 9.1), further circles are drawn over the middle of the femur and tibia so that angular, rotational and translational deformities can be recorded diagrammatically. The boxes labelled V and H are used to record respectively

TECHNICAL ANALYSIS FORM   **LOWER LIMB**

Name _____ No. _____ Age _____ Sex _____

Date of Onset _____ Cause _____

Occupation _____ Present Lower-Limb Equipment _____

Diagnosis _____

_____

Ambulatory ☐   Non-Ambulatory ☐

MAJOR IMPAIRMENTS:

A. Skeletal
    1. Bone and Joints: Normal ☐   Abnormal _____
    2. Ligaments: Normal ☐   Abnormal ☐   Knee: AC ☐   PC ☐   MC ☐   LC ☐
                                                      Ankle: MC ☐   LC ☐

    3. Extremity Shortening: None ☐   Left ☐   Right ☐
        Amount of Discrepancy: A.S.S.-Heel _____   A.S.S.-MTP _____   MTP-Heel _____

B. Sensation: Normal ☐   Abnormal ☐
    1. Anaesthesia ☐   Hypaesthesia ☐   Location: _____
        Protective Sensation: Retained ☐   Lost ☐
    2. Pain ☐   Location: _____

C. Skin: Normal ☐   Abnormal: _____

D. Vascular: Normal ☐   Abnormal ☐   Right ☐   Left ☐

E. Balance: Normal ☐   Impaired ☐   Support: _____

F. Gait Deviations: _____
    _____

G. Other Impairments: _____

─────────────────────────── **LEGEND** ───────────────────────────

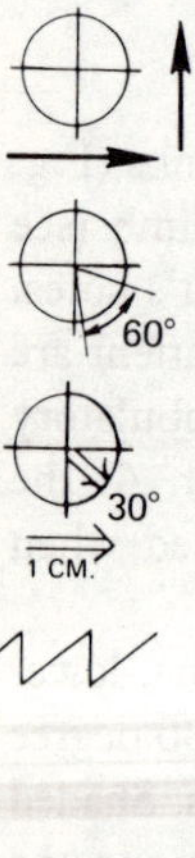

⊕ ↑ = Direction of Translatory Motion

= Abnormal Degree of Rotary Motion 60°

= Fixed Position 30° 1 CM.

∿ = Fracture

Volitional Force (V)
N = Normal
G = Good
F = Fair
P = Poor
T = Trace
Z = Zero

Hypertonic Muscle (H)
N = Normal
M = Mild
Mo = Moderate
S = Severe

Proprioception (P)
N = Normal
I = Impaired
A = Absent
D = Local Distension or Enlargement

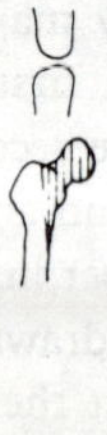

= Pseudarthrosis

= Absence of Segment

Fig. 9.1

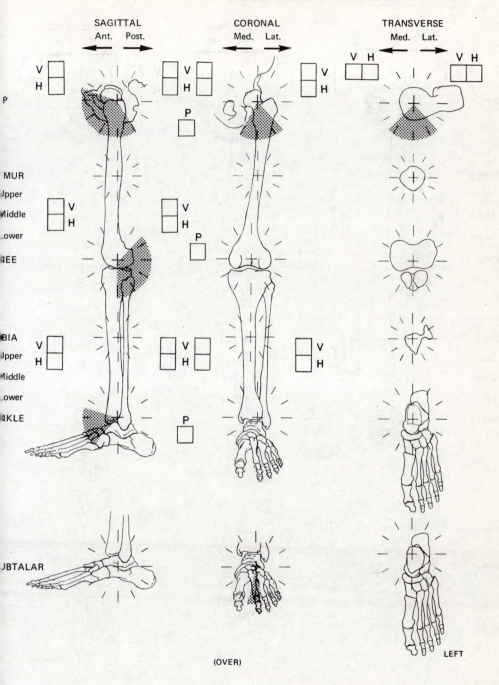

Fig. 9.1

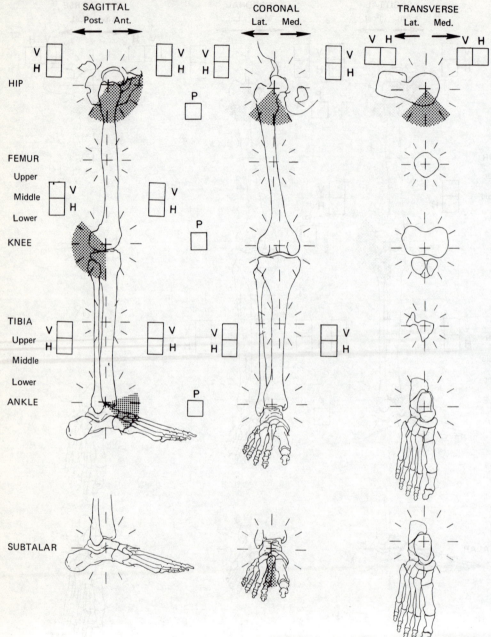

Fig. 9.1

Summary of Functional Disability _____

_____

_____

_____

_____

Treatment Objectives:

Prevent/Correct Deformity ☐	Improve Ambulation ☐	
Reduce Axial Load ☐	Fracture Treatment ☐	
Protect Joint ☐	Other_____	

ORTHOTIC RECOMMENDATION

LOWER LIMB		FLEX	EXT	ABD	ADD .	ROTATION Int.	ROTATION Ext.	AXIAL LOAD
HKAO	Hip							
KAO	Thigh							
	Knee							
AFO	Leg							
	Ankle	(Dorsi)	(Plantar)					
	Subtalar					(Inver.)	(Ever.)	
FO Foot	Midtarsal							
	Met.-phal.							

REMARKS:

_____

Signature   Date

_____

KEY: Use the following symbols to indicate desired control of designated function:

F = FREE   — Free motion.
A = ASSIST   — Application of an external force for the purpose of increasing the range, velocity, or force of a motion.
R = RESIST   — Application of an external force for the purpose of decreasing the velocity or force of a motion.
S = STOP   — Inclusion of a static unit to deter an undesired motion in one direction.
v = Variable   — A unit that can be adjusted without making a structural change.
H = HOLD   — Elimination of all motion in prescribed plane (verify position).
L = LOCK   — Device includes an optional lock.

Fig. 9.1

the voluntary power and degree of hypertonicity of each muscle group. The box labelled P is for recording proprioception.

The fourth page has spaces for recording a summary of the functional disability and treatment objectives. Also on this page is the orthotic recommendation along with a key for its use.

Detailed instructions for the use of the technical analysis forms and illustrated cases for practice in using them are to be found in the *Atlas of Orthotics* (1975).

TERMINOLOGY FOR ORTHOSES

As well as designing technical analysis forms, it was also necessary to develop a logical terminology for orthoses with which a physician could communicate to an orthotist or prosthetist the function desired from a device (Harris, 1973). It was decided to consider that the body consisted of three major anatomical regions, upper limbs, lower limbs and the spine; that all proper names would be eliminated from the terminology; and that orthoses would be described by the joints which they encompassed.

The three major anatomical regions of the body are divided as follows:

Table 9.1

Upper limb		Lower limb		Spine	
S	Shoulder (Humerus)	H	Hip (Thigh)	C	Cervical
E	Elbow (Forearm)	K	Knee (Leg)	T	Thoracic
W	Wrist	A	Ankle	L	Lumbar (Lumbo-sacral)
H	Hand	F	Foot Subtalar	SI	Sacroiliac
	Fingers MP		Midtarsal		
	2–5 PIP		Met.-phal.		
	DIP				
	Thumb CM				
	MP				
	IP				

The terminology accepts the joint complexes of the hand, wrist and foot as individual descriptive units. Sometimes, for certain prescriptions, it may be necessary to subdivide these units into their component joints.

The areas listed in brackets are not part of the basic system, but are a modification which permits the system to be used in fracture bracing and other situations, where an orthosis does not cross a joint. As the use of the full names is unwieldly, the initial letters are used. A long-leg caliper supporting the knee, ankle and foot therefore becomes a KAFO or knee-ankle-foot orthosis.

After indicating the site of the orthosis in terms of the joints which are encompassed by the orthosis, it is necessary to specify what action the orthosis should have on these joints. The movements which may occur at normal and pathological joints are flexion, extension, abduction, adduction and rotation. In addition joints and long bones may be subjected to axial loading. Other terms are used when these are more familiar in relation to certain regions, for example pronation and supination instead of rotation of the forearm; lateral flexion of the spine to the left and right instead of abduction; inversion and eversion instead of rotation of the foot; and opposition of the thumb.

By arranging the joints vertically and the possible movements at these joints horizontally, orthotic recommendation charts for the three major regions of the body can be compiled. On these charts, movements at joints which can occur only with pathological conditions, are blocked out.

Each of the movements possible at a joint can be controlled in five ways (see below). Some controls may be variable or be capable of being locked in position. The range of permitted movement is specified in degrees, and the permitted axial loading as a percentage of normal load. The controls are as follows:

F Free — Free movement

A Assist — Application of an external force to increase the range, velocity or force of a movement

R Resist — Application of an external force to decrease the velocity or force of a movement

S Stop — The inclusion of a static unit to prevent undesired movement in a specified direction. When used alone, S means the restraint of gross movement in the neutral position of the joint

H Hold — Elimination of all movement in a specified plane. The joint is held in a specified position

V Variable — The control can be adjusted by the patient or the orthotist, without making any structural change to the orthosis. It is seldom used except with 'STOP'

L Lock — The orthosis can be locked in position

The terminology thus covers the site and extent of the orthosis, the direction in which movements at joints are permitted or prevented, and the way in which these movements are controlled.

This system should enable the doctor to identify clearly the biomechanical defects and to describe his intentions, and also should leave the orthotist free to make the best interpretation of these intentions with regard to the type of splint, fittings and materials most suited to the patient's needs.

Although the new terminology enables a clear anatomical and mechanical description to be given of the aims of the orthosis, it cannot itself describe the particular pattern of the appliance which the doctor may know from his experience to be best suited to the patient's needs. It is long-winded in its description of commonly used and familiar appliances, in that a drop foot splint becomes an AFO–dorsi A–plantar R (ankle-foot orthosis – dorsiflexion assist – plantar flexion resist); a mallet finger splint becomes HO–DIP–H extension (hand orthosis – distal interphalangeal joint – hold in extension); and a Milwaukee brace becomes a CTLSO (cervical-thoracic-lumbar-sacroiliac orthosis) with 28 control symbols (Harris, 1973). The system is suited to the situation where there is not a commonly used orthosis which will fulfill the patient's needs and where the orthotist is comprehensively trained and experienced.

There is still a great deal to be said in favour of a prescription written in general terms and backed up by personal contact with the orthotist.

A sample prescription in general terms is given below for a child who contracted poliomyelitis which affected one of his lower limbs, leaving weakness particularly of extension of the knee and dorsiflexion of the ankle. Contractures of the joints have not developed.

Name	John Smith
Age	13 years
Diagnosis	Poliomyelitis right lower limb with weakness of the quadriceps and dorsiflexors of the ankle. Orthosis required to stabilise the knee and compensate for weakness of dorsiflexion of the ankle
Rx	Right long leg orthosis with cuff top, adjustable side bars, double automatic ring lock knee joints, round spur pieces and heel sockets with posterior heel stops, anterior thigh pad, calf band and ankle strap

CHECKING AN ORTHOSIS

After the patient has received his orthosis, it must be checked by the prescribing doctor. In the case of an orthosis for the lower limb, the following must be checked.

General

— Does the orthosis correspond to the prescription?
— Is the orthosis of adequate strength and rigidity?
— Is the orthosis free of sharp edges and rough areas?
— Does the patient find the orthosis comfortable, functional and satisfactory in appearance?
— Does it operate quietly?
— Can the patient sit comforably when wearing it?
— When the orthosis is removed, is the skin free of any sign of irritation?

Footwear

— Does the shoe or boot fit satisfactorily when the sole and heel are flat on the ground?
— Is any insert comfortable, and is it held in place firmly?
— Are any adaptations to the shoe or boot those that were ordered?
— Is a T-strap, if fitted, attached to the shoe or boot correctly, is it comfortable and does it give adequate support?
— Do the heel stops, if fitted, make contact simultaneously with the side-bars?

Side-bars

— Are the side-bars lying in the mid-lateral line of the limb, and are they contoured to the shape of the limb, with adequate clearance of bony prominences such as the head of the fibula?

— If the orthosis is for a child, are the side-bars adjustable for length?

— Is there clearance between the top of the inner side-bar and the perineum?

— Is the top of the outer side-bar just below the tip of the greater trochanter, and at least 1 inch (2.5 cm) above the top of the inner side-bar.

— Are the joints aligned with the anatomical joints, and do they provide the desired range of movement?

— Are the locks secure and easy to operate?

— Are the thigh and calf bands of the proper width, contoured to the shape of the limb and correctly sited?

— If the orthosis is designed to decrease axial loading, is the reduction adequate at the heel?

TRAINING IN THE USE OF AN ORTHOSIS

When a patient receives an orthosis, it is essential that he understands the function of the orthosis, how to put it on and take it off, and how to look after it. In addition he may require training in the use of the orthosis, to enable him to acquire the maximum benefit from its use.

The training which a patient requires and receives is determined by his general medical condition, and is carried out by trained staff under close medical supervision. Before walking in an orthosis, the patient must be able to balance, initially on both feet and then on each foot separately. Exercises to strengthen certain groups of muscles may be required before the patient even wears his orthosis. Walking aids or even parallel bars may be necessary initially. When walking is started, it is important that strides of equal length are taken even if these are very small initially. As confidence and strength improve, the strides can be lengthened.

Once the patient can walk with confidence, he must be taught to walk up and down inclines, and to climb up and down steps. It is important also that the patient can sit down in and rise up from different types and height of chair, including a wheelchair if appropriate, as well as the toilet and car. Whenever possible patients should be taught how to pick objects up from the floor, and how to kneel, sit and lie on the floor and how to get up again.

HOW TO LOOK AFTER AN ORTHOSIS

Every patient who wears an orthosis must be instructed in its care, and must be advised to:

— Always handle the orthosis with care, and to avoid dropping it.

— Examine his skin every night for evidence of undue pressure from the orthosis.

— Each week open all locks and remove any accumulated dirt or fluff.

— Oil each joint weekly.

— Inspect all moving parts for wear, and ensure that all bolts and screws are present and not loose.

— Inspect all leather parts regularly, keep them in good condition, and get any necessary repairs carried out immediately.

— Keep the heels and soles of the footwear in good condition.

REFERENCES

Harris, E.E. (1973) A new orthotics terminology. A guide to its use for prescription and fee schedules. *Orthotics and Prosthetics*, **27**, 2.

The Committee on Prosthetics and Orthotics, American Academy of Orthopaedic Surgeons. (1975) *The Atlas of Orthotics*. St Louis: Mosby.

10.

Spinal orthoses

Over the years many spinal orthoses have been designed and later modified. This development has occurred largely in the absence of detailed knowledge of the biomechanics of the spine, with the result that the value, in mechanical terms, of many orthoses is doubtful. Much work is being done on the biomechanics of the normal spine, but as yet little on the effect of spinal orthoses on function in either the normal or diseased spine. This work must be increased so that orthoses which limit the different movements occurring in the different regions of the spine can be designed, manufactured and prescribed with precision. Before spinal orthoses can be prescribed, knowledge of the functional anatomy of the spine is essential. It must be remembered, however, that the movements which occur in a particular region of the normal spine may differ from those which may be possible in the presence of disease.

FUNCTIONAL ANATOMY OF THE SPINE

MOVEMENTS OCCURRING IN THE DIFFERENT REGIONS OF THE SPINE

The spinal column is basically a segmented cylindrical structure which subserves three main functions: protection of the spinal cord, support of the trunk, and transmission of the weight of the head, upper limbs and trunk to the pelvis and lower limbs. The segmental nature of the vertebral column confers considerable mobility upon the spine by the summation of the small amounts of movement that can occur between the individual segments.

The movements that occur in the spine are forward flexion, extension, lateral flexion and rotation. The range of movement and the directions in which it can occur differ in each region of the spine, depending upon the anatomical structure of that region.

Cervical spine
In the cervical region the range of forward flexion, extension and lateral flexion is considerable. Rotation mainly occurs between the atlas and axis. Below the

level of the axis, the configuration of the articular facets prevents rotation occurring between the individual cervical vertebrae (C2 to C7) without concomitant lateral flexion.

Thoracic spine

In the thoracic region, the ribs limit rotation less than they limit movements in the other directions. Up to 6 degrees of rotation can occur between adjacent vertebrae (Gregersen and Lucas, 1967). The centre of axial rotation in the thoracic region lies within or anterior to the intervertebral disc. Lateral flexion in this region is accompanied by some degree of rotation.

Lumbar spine

In the lumbar region, forward flexion, extension and lateral flexion are free, but rotation is limited not so much by the configuration of the articular facets of the posterior articulations as by the annulus fibrosus which restricts lateral displacement of adjacent vertebral bodies. The centre of axial rotation in the lumbar region lies posterior to the articular processes. Up to 10 degrees of rotation can occur at the thoraco-lumbar junction. A further 10 degrees of rotation can occur between the first and fifth lumbar vertebrae in the sitting position, this being increased to 16 degrees in the standing position (Gregersen and Lucas, 1967). Approximately 6 degrees of rotation, which is always associated with flexion of the fifth lumbar vertebra on the sacrum, can occur at the lumbo-sacral junction (Lumsden and Morris, 1968).

During walking, the pelvis and shoulders rotate in opposite directions, the amount of rotation depending upon the length of each step.

The range of lateral flexion is greater in the upper region of the lumbar spine than in the lower, being maximal at the L3/4 level (Tanz, 1953), whereas the range of forward flexion is greater in the lower region of the lumbar spine than in the upper, being maximal at the L4/5 and L5/S1 levels (Tanz, 1953; Allbrook, 1957). In forward flexion from the standing position, movement occurs both in the lumbar spine and at the hip joints. The distance, therefore, between the finger tips and the floor, on carrying out this manoeuvre varies from one individual to another depending upon the length of the hamstring muscles and the mobility of the lumbar spine. For this reason, the range of lumbar flexion should be tested in both the standing and sitting positions. The lumbar spine is substantially flexed when sitting erect, and the flexion is increased markedly when sitting slumped, the degree of forward flexion between the fourth and fifth lumbar vertebrae actually exceeding that observed during maximal forward bending (Norton and Brown, 1957). As movement of the lumbar spine largely occurs secondary to movements of the lower limbs on the trunk (Troup et al, 1968), absolute immobilisation of the lumbar spine cannot be achieved by external support without severely restricting the movements of the lower limbs.

During forward flexion and the early stages of extension of the *flexed* trunk, especially if this action is associated with lifting, considerable forces are generated within the spine, particularly in the lumbo-sacral region. Contraction of the thoracic and abdominal muscles and those of the diaphragm and pelvic floor, raises the pressures within the thoracic and abdominal cavities and converts these cavities into rigid-walled structures, which are capable of transmitting forces produced during bending and lifting, and thereby reducing the forces within the spine (Davis, 1956; Bartelink, 1957). The pressures within the thoracic and abdominal cavities increase as the weight lifted increases (Davis and Troup, 1964). It is calculated that these pressures decrease the force on the lumbo-sacral disc by 30 per cent and on the lower thoracic spine by 50 per cent (Morris et al, 1961). The mechanical advantage of the pressure increases is greatest when the lumbar spine is flexed. These pressure increases thus have their greatest effect during the acceleration phase of lifting before the spine begins to extend (Davis and Troup, 1965).

The load on the intervertebral discs in the lumbar region depends upon the position of the trunk and the weight of the body above but largely upon the tension developed by the muscles of the trunk. The pressures within these discs are greatest in the sitting position and are reduced by 30 per cent on standing and by 50 per cent on reclining (Nachemson and Morris, 1964).

ORTHOSES FOR THE THORACIC AND LUMBAR SPINES

FUNCTION OF SPINAL ORTHOSES

The many different spinal orthoses which have been designed can be divided into two groups, supportive and corrective. They are used to relieve pain, to support weakened or paralysed muscles and unstable joints, to immobilise the vertebral column in the best functional position while healing occurs, to prevent the occurrence of deformity, and to correct an existing deformity. The supportive group includes orthoses made from various fabrics (belts and corsets), rigid spinal braces, and those moulded from leather, plastic, plaster-of-Paris and Plastazote. Those orthoses in the corrective group produce an active corrective force in one or more directions. The various functional advantages that have been claimed for these different appliances are difficult to evaluate.

Investigations have been carried out in an attempt to determine the effect of various spinal supports upon the mobility of the spine. However, the results of these investigations may not be applicable to patients suffering from disorders of the spine as the observations were made upon people with normal spines.

Fabric supports restrict only the extremes of forward flexion and extension (Van Leuven and Troup, 1969), and have a variable and unpredictable effect upon rotation at the lumbo-sacral junction (Lumsden and Morris, 1968).

An inflated corset can reduce the pressure within the lumbar discs when standing (Nachemson and Morris, 1964). These findings may not be applicable to the fabric supports prescribed for patients.

Long spinal braces, for example the Taylor brace (see below), and the plaster-of-Paris moulded spinal support, increase movement at the lumbo-sacral junction, but decrease movement at the upper levels (Norton and Brown, 1957).

Rotation at the lumbo-sacral junction is restricted by short spinal braces when standing, but increased when walking (Lumsden and Morris, 1968).

In spite of the apparent mechanical deficiencies of spinal supports many patients obtain symptomatic relief from their use. This relief may be psychological, or may result from abdominal compression, from support of a pendulous abdomen and a concomitant decrease in lumbar lordosis, from a change in the amount of movement occurring in different regions of the spine, from a decrease in activity of the various associated muscle groups, from local support of the sacro-iliac joints and ilio-lumbar ligaments or from a combination of all these factors. It is interesting that subjective support can be obtained by the application of non-elastic adhesive strapping to the lumbar and gluteal regions of the back.

SUPPORTIVE SPINAL ORTHOSES

Fabric spinal orthoses (spinal belts and corsets)

Spinal belts and corsets are the most commonly prescribed spinal orthoses (Perry, 1970). The majority of these orthoses are made from jean (twilled weave Egyptian cotton), coutil (herring-bone weave Egyptian cotton) or canvas (plain weave American cotton). They can be made also from duck (light canvas), rayon, nylon or airtex (open weave cotton). They are reinforced as necessary with bone or metal strips. Corsets extend further down over the buttocks and upper thighs than do belts to give a smoother contour, and therefore are prescribed for women. Belts are prescribed for men.

These orthoses encircle the sacral region and extend a variable distance upwards, the term applied to them (sacro-iliac, lumbo-sacral, thoraco-lumbar) depending upon their depth posteriorly (see below). In front they are fastened with straps and buckles, eyelets and laces or hooks and eyes. In addition a fulcrum strap (Figs. 10.1 and 10.2), broad posteriorly where it is attached to the mid-line, and narrowing towards the front, fastens in the front with a buckle. Elastic insets may be let into the upper and lower margins to ease the fitting over the costal margin and around the buttocks respectively.

Fabric orthoses, even when reinforced with metal strips, do not immobilise the spine; they only restrict the extremes of forward and lateral flexion, and extension. They probably function by supplying subjective support and by reminding the patient to avoid movements which may bring on or exacerbate his symptoms.

A sacroiliac orthosis (SIO)

This is 2–6 inches (5–15 cm) deep posteriorly and basically consists of a wide belt of leather or fabric which encircles the pelvis, passing between the greater trochanters and the iliac crests on each side. It is fastened anteriorly by straps and buckles or hooks. Perineal straps may be added to prevent the support from riding upwards.

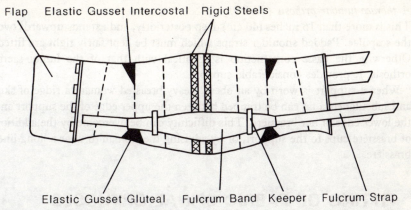

Flap   Elastic Gusset Intercostal   Rigid Steels

Elastic Gusset Gluteal   Fulcrum Band   Keeper   Fulcrum Strap

Fig.10.1 Lumbo-sacral orthosis. Typical minimum depth at the centre back is that from the thoraco-lumbar junction to the middle of the sacrum.

A lumbo-sacral orthosis (LSO) (Figs 10.1, 10.2)

This is 8–16 inches (20–40 cm) deep posteriorly. It extends up to the thoraco-lumbar junction posteriorly and covers the entire abdomen anteriorly. It has a closely fitting fulcrum strap, attached posteriorly, which passes around the pelvis between the greater trochanters and the iliac crests and buckles firmly in the region of the symphysis pubis, thus obtaining a grip on the pelvis and giving a stable foundation to the support. Flexible or rigid vertical metal strips are incorporated posteriorly on each side of the spinous processes to reinforce the support and to provide a wide stable area posteriorly from which the support can act on the abdomen. Further vertical metal strips can be added to increase rigidity. To ease pressure on the costal margin, elastic gussets can be let into the upper edge. Perineal straps or suspenders may be fitted to prevent the support from riding upwards. The support is adjusted by straps and buckles or eyelets and laces. A 'quick release' panel of hooks and eyes is often incorporated.

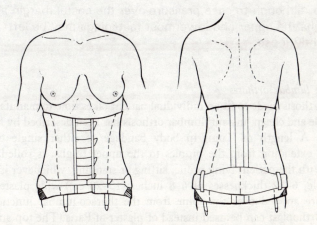

Fig. 10.2 Lumbo-sacral orthosis can be fitted with suspenders or groin straps.

A thoraco-lumbar orthosis (TLSO)

This is more than 16 inches (40 cm) deep posteriorly, and extends upwards over the scapulae. Padded shoulder straps which must be kept fairly tight are fitted. Otherwise the basic construction is identical with that of the lumbo-sacral orthosis. It provides considerable support.

When a support is worn by an obese, heavy-breasted woman, a ridge of skin and subcutaneous fat can be trapped between the upper edge of the support and the lower edge of her brassière. This difficulty can be overcome by the addition of brassière cups to the support, or by advising the woman to wear a 'long-line' brassière.

FITTING OF FABRIC SPINAL ORTHOSES

Check the orthosis

- The orthosis must be adequate for its intended function.
- It must extend well down to the symphysis pubis.
- It must fit firmly and smoothly over the greater trochanters, iliac crests and buttocks.
- The posterior steel strips must follow closely the curves of the sacrum and spine.
- It must not interfere with hip flexion and sitting.
- It must not ride upwards.
- It must be comfortable. Some patients who have not worn an orthosis before may find it uncomfortable at first. They should be advised to gradually lengthen the time they wear it, as they would do with new shoes.

Instruct the patient

- The fulcrum strap must always be firmly buckled.
- The other abdominal straps or laces must be tightened firmly also, although to ease pressure over the costal margin and thighs the upper and lowermost fastenings may be left slightly loose.

Immediate lumbar orthoses

A fabric orthosis made to fit an individual patient takes time to manufacture. An easily made and cheap 'instant' lumbar orthosis has been described by Nichols et al (1966). A length of Tubigrip body bandage of either single or double thickness, extending from the nipples to the upper thighs, is rolled onto the patient. With the patient lying prone, sitting or standing, whichever is the most comfortable, 6–12 thicknesses of 6–8 inches (15–20 cm) wide plaster-of-Paris bandage are applied over the spine from the thoraco-lumbar junction to the sacrum. Orthoplast can be used instead of plaster-of-Paris. The top and bottom of the Tubigrip bandage are turned back and fixed down.

Rigid spinal orthoses

All rigid spinal orthoses, except the anterior hyperextension orthosis described later, are constructed on the basis of a metal frame which takes firm support from the pelvis. Metal uprights, joined together by various cross bars, are attached to the pelvic support. Devices to apply pressure over the abdomen and over the front of the shoulders are provided. The metal frame is padded with felt and covered with leather.

The metal frame must have a firm foundation on the pelvis to hold the appliance in contact with the body, and to distribute the body weight, transmitted by the uprights, over a large area. This can be obtained by using a pelvic band or a moulded pelvic corset. A pelvic band is made from flat metal bars which encircle the posterior and lateral aspects of the pelvis and press upon the sacrum. These metal bars extend for a variable distance towards the midline anteriorly in different types of braces. A moulded pelvic corset (Fig. 10.8) gives a firm grip around the pelvis. The corset may be made of leather or plastic. A negative cast of the pelvis and abdomen is taken with plaster-of-Paris or Plastazote, from which a positive plaster model is made. The leather or plastic is moulded over the plaster model.

The metal uprights attached to the pelvic support extend upwards for varying distances depending upon the length of spine to be supported. There are two uprights posteriorly lying on each side of the spinous processes — the back lever. To obtain more rigidity, further uprights can be attached laterally or anteriorly.

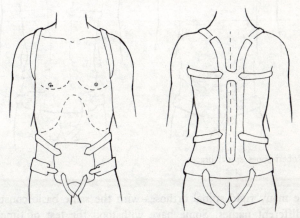

Fig. 10.3   Taylor spinal brace.

The uprights are joined together by horizontal cross bars. When lateral or anterior uprights are present, the cross bar in the thoracic region extends anteriorly around the trunk below the axillae (Fig. 10.4).

Abdominal support is obtained by an abdominal plate (Figs 10.3, 10.5) attached by straps and buckles to the metal frame, or by a fabric corset (Fig. 10.4). Pressure over the front of the shoulders to hold them back into the brace can be obtained by using padded shoulder straps or clavicular pads which curve upwards and press on the chest wall in the infra-clavicular region.

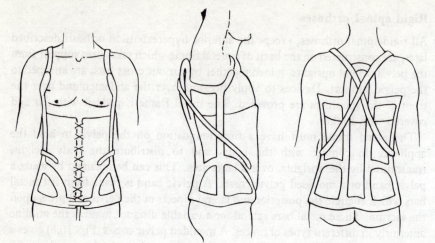

Fig. 10.4 Fisher spinal brace.

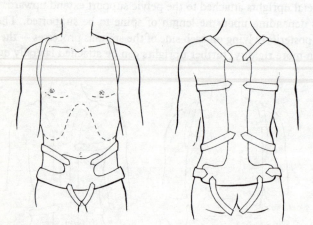

Fig. 10.5 Robert Jones spinal brace.

There are many rigid spinal orthoses with the same basic construction but called by different names. Some have withstood the test of time, while the existence of others is perpetuated by the written word (Perry, 1970). Described below are some of the more commonly used rigid spinal orthoses. The descriptions used are those found in the Surgical Appliances Contract 1972 of the Department of Health and Social Security.

Taylor spinal brace (TLSO) (Fig. 10.3)
In 1863, C.F. Taylor described a spinal brace, for use in the treatment of tuberculosis of the spine, which can be considered as the prototype of all spinal orthoses designed to support the thoraco-lumbar spine. It consists of a wide

straight spring-steel pelvic band which extends forward in front of the anterior superior iliac spines. The pelvic band is completed anteriorly with leather straps and buckles. There are two parallel posterior uprights connected at the level of the scapulae by a cross bar made from a thin plate of moulded steel. Above this level the uprights gently angle outwards towards the shoulders. The steel frame is padded with a thin layer of felt and covered with leather.

Shoulder straps, covered by upward extensions of the leather covering the posterior uprights, pass from the uprights over the shoulders and back under the axillae to be attached to the cross bar. Abdominal support is provided by a rigid, padded, leather abdominal plate, extending between the umbilicus and the symphysis pubis, which is attached below to the pelvic band and above to the posterior uprights by two straps which pass backwards around the loins. Groin straps are fitted also.

The Taylor brace limits forward flexion, extension and lateral flexion of the thoraco-lumbar region of the spine and, to some extent, rotation of the lumbar and lower thoracic regions of the spine. It increases movement at the lumbo-sacral junction (Norton and Brown, 1957).

Fisher spinal brace (TLSO) (Fig. 10.4)

The Fisher spinal brace was described originally in 1886. It consists of a metal pelvic band to which two metal pelvic hoops, one on each side, are attached. These pelvic hoops arch over the iliac crests. There are two posterior uprights and two adjustable lateral uprights. A transverse metal bar, at the level of the inferior angles of the scapulae, joins the posterior and lateral uprights and ends anteriorly in axillary crutches. All the metal parts except the lateral uprights are padded with a thin layer of felt and covered with leather.

Abdominal support is provided by a fabric corset which extends forward from the lateral uprights and fastens in the mid-line anteriorly. Well padded shoulder straps pass up from the tips of the axillary crutches, over the shoulders, cross posteriorly, and then swing forwards again to buckle on the front of the corset on each side level with the iliac crests.

The axillary crutches are not designed to bear weight. If they press into the axillae, nerve palsies will result.

The Fisher spinal brace limits forward flexion and extension of the lower thoracic and upper lumbar regions of the spine. Lateral flexion is limited more than with the Taylor spinal brace. Rotation of the thoracic spine is limited also.

Thomas or Jones spinal brace (TLSO) (Fig. 10.5)

This type of spinal brace was designed originally by H.O. Thomas. It was used extensively by Sir Robert Jones instead of a plaster-of-Paris moulded support, for the ambulant treatment of spinal tuberculosis (Jones and Lovett, 1923).

It consists of a large padded pelvic strap which is attached posteriorly to a padded, leather-covered metal frame. Abdominal support is provided by an abdominal pad to which are buckled waist, pelvic and groin straps. Shoulder straps pass from the metal frame over the shoulders and under the axillae to be reattached to the metal frame at the level of the inferior angles of the scapulae.

FITTING OF RIGID SPINAL ORTHOSES

— Tighten the pelvic band and ensure that the pelvic band or pelvic corset fits snugly around the pelvis.
— Check that the posterior metal uprights follow closely the contour of the spine.
— After checking the posterior uprights, tighten the shoulder straps if fitted.
— Fasten the groin and waist straps, abdominal plate or fabric corset if fitted.
— Check that the axillary crutches, if fitted, do not press into the axillae.
— With a Jones spinal brace, when the patient stands with a good posture, it should be possible to slip two fingers between the back lever and the upper part of the spine.

Anterior hyperextension spinal brace (TLSO) (Fig. 10.6)

This type of brace utilises a completely different method of construction from the above spinal braces. It was described originally by Hoadley in 1896, who used it to provide mechanical support 'of the spinal column between the middle of the lumbar and the middle of the thoracic regions'. It employs the principle of three-point action of a bending force. Numerous modifications to this brace have been made, but that of Baker (1942) is described here.

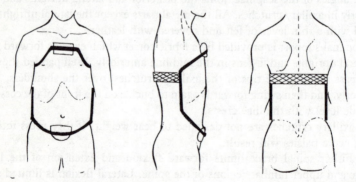

Fig. 10.6 Anterior hyperextension brace.

The anterior hyperextension spinal brace consists basically of a rectangular metal frame, the short sides of which fit over the front of the thorax and abdomen, in the pectoral and inguinal regions respectively, while the longer sides lie in the mid-axillary line. Pads, hinged on the metal frame, lie over the pubis and upper sternum. An elastic strap passes posteriorly from the side arms over the thoracic spine and is kept sufficiently tight to hold the brace against the patient's body. Additional pelvic and thoracic straps may be added to keep the brace in position.

Moulded spinal orthoses

Moulded spinal orthoses fit the contours of the trunk and distribute the body weight over a very large area. They can be made from leather, plastic, plaster-of-Paris, Plastazote*, or the recently introduced Neofract* system. Their rigidity will depend upon the material used in their construction. A leather support can be reinforced by attaching metal bands. A Plastazote support is less rigid than a plaster-of-Paris or plastic support, but it is light and comfortable to wear, and can be moulded directly onto the patient, as can plaster-of-Paris. Leather and plastic supports require to be moulded over a positive model of the patient and therefore are more expensive and take longer to make than do those made from plaster-of-Paris or Plastazote.

These supports must extend from the symphysis pubis to the upper sternum anteriorly and be accurately fitted around the pelvis. They are cut low posteriorly (Fig. 10.7).

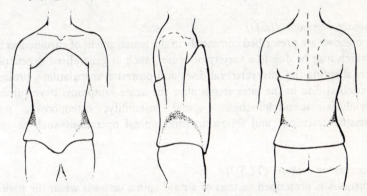

Fig. 10.7 Moulded spinal jacket, extends from the upper sternum to the symphysis pubis anteriorly and is cut lower posteriorly.

PRESCRIBING A SUPPORTIVE SPINAL ORTHOSIS

It is impossible here to give detailed indications for the prescription of the various spinal orthoses, as they depend upon the underlying spinal disability and its site and extent, the intensity of the patient's symptoms and their response to other forms of treatment, the patient's age and sex, whether the appliance is to be worn permanently or only for a limited time, and the function required of the appliance (Berger, 1969).

Before a spinal orthosis is prescribed, it is imperative that an accurate history is taken, a detailed physical and radiological examination is performed, and other special investigations are carried out in an attempt to diagnose accurately the cause and site of the patient's symptoms. Treatment in all cases must be directed towards the underlying cause of the symptoms which often may be relieved by means other than a spinal orthosis. When symptoms persist or change, in spite of apparent adequate treatment, the patient must be reassessed carefully, as the symptoms may be due to a pathological condition, for example tuberculosis or neoplasia, which could not be detected initially.

---

*See Appendix

Spinal orthoses are prescribed commonly under a proper name, which name may be that of the original designer or someone who has modified the appliance. In addition many appliances, although called by the same proper name, may differ considerably in construction from place to place, and appliances of the same design and construction may be called by different names in different places. It is important therefore to describe accurately the orthosis required, the movements which it is intended to control, and to ensure that the orthosis supplied to the patient fits correctly and fulfils its intended function.

Fabric spinal orthoses

Sacroiliac orthosis (SIO)
This orthosis may be prescribed for the rare cases of sacroiliac strain or instability of the symphysis pubis.

Lumbo-sacral orthosis (LSO)
These orthoses are prescribed commonly in the management of chronic low back pain which may be due to a variety of causes, such as generalised degenerative changes affecting the intervertebral discs and posterior articulations, prolapsed intervertebral disc in the later stages after the acute symptoms have subsided, spondylolysis, spondylolisthesis, spinal instability, osteoporosis, minor compression fractures, and following some spinal operations such as spinal fusion.

Thoraco-lumbar orthosis (TLSO)
This orthosis is prescribed instead of a rigid spinal orthosis when the patient's symptoms arise from the thoracic or upper lumbar regions of the spine, from conditions such as generalised degenerative changes, senile kyphosis, osteoporosis, minor compression fractures, and spinal infections in the elderly.

Rigid spinal orthoses

Rigid spinal orthoses are more effective in reducing movement in the lower thoracic and upper lumbar regions of the spine than fabric supports. It must be remembered, however, that movement in the adjacent regions of the spine, especially the lumbo-sacral junction, tends to be increased (Norton and Brown, 1957), and this increase in movement may give rise to pain, particularly if degenerative changes are present.

Fisher, Taylor and Jones spinal braces
All these spinal orthoses limit, to some degree, forward flexion, extension, lateral flexion and rotation in the thoraco-lumbar region of the spine, the Fisher spinal brace being the most effective, and the Jones the least. These spinal braces are used in the ambulant management of tuberculosis of the lower thoracic and upper lumbar regions of the spine, the more severe vertebral compression fractures, vertebral osteochondritis and osteoporosis, and marked weakness of the trunk musculature.

Anterior hyperextension spinal brace
This brace is uncomfortable if the pressure exerted over the thoracic spine is too great. It was designed to provide extension, but is more comfortable when used merely to prevent excessive forward flexion. Conditions which can be treated with this brace are compression fractures of the vertebral bodies and ankylosing spondylitis.

Moulded spinal orthoses
Moulded leather or plastic spinal orthoses are reserved usually for the management of severe deformities of the spine from any cause for which it would be impossible to manufacture and fit a fabric or rigid spinal orthosis.

Moulded spinal supports of plaster-of-Paris or Plastazote are used when the need for a support is temporary.

CORRECTIVE SPINAL ORTHOSES

Milwaukee brace (CTLSO) (Fig. 10.8)
The Milwaukee brace (Blount et al, 1958) is an active corrective spinal orthosis used almost exclusively in the ambulant treatment of structural scoliosis, the aim being to postpone, temporarily or permanently, the need for operation. It

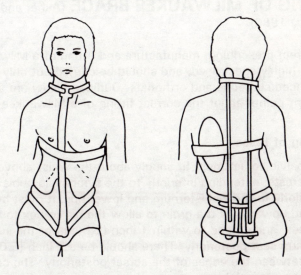

Fig. 10.8 Milwaukee brace. Note the throat mould anteriorly and the two occipital pads posteriorly.

frequently has to be worn for a number of years, until the spine is stable. It is used also in the post-operative period. This brace is used occasionally in the management of ankylosing spondylitis and tuberculosis or other infection of the upper thoracic region of the spine. In these later instances, a pressure pad (see below) is not necessary.

It consists of a moulded leather or Ortholene pelvic corset which fits snugly over the iliac crests, around the waist, and curves upward in front to support the abdomen. It is cut lower at the sides to avoid pressure on the costal margin. Metal side bars are attached to the leather pelvic corset to form a base from which one anterior and two posterior metal uprights pass upwards to a ring around the neck. This ring is inclined at 20 degrees to the horizontal, being lower anteriorly. The uprights are adjustable to allow for growth. There is a throat mould anteriorly. This replaces the previous submental pad, and its use avoids hypoplasia of the mandible and adverse effects upon the teeth. The throat mould does not press on the mandible, but closely follows the contour of the throat at the level of the hyoid, without pressing on the larynx. There are two occipital pads posteriorly.

Rib rotation is corrected by a pressure pad located over the rib prominences. The pressure pad is fixed to a single, heavy, broad leather strap which is attached to the uprights at the desired level by stud fastenings. The leather strap is passed over the posterior bar on the convex side so that the pressure is applied directly from the lateral side. To avoid pressure on a breast, the leather strap can be attached to an outrigger on the anterior bar.

Because of the close moulding of the pelvic corset, the brace has to be remade as growth occurs.

FITTING OF MILWAUKEE BRACE (Asher and Whitney, 1980)

The correct prescribing, manufacture and fitting of a Milwaukee brace is highly specialised, and should be carried out only by experienced surgeons and orthotists. Outlined below are some important points about the correct fitting of a Milwaukee brace.

Checking of brace

— The pelvic corset must fit snugly about the waist above the iliac crests, extending inferiorly to the symphysis pubis and superiorly to the xiphisternum and lower ribs. It must be curved upwards at the groin to allow the hip to flex to 90 degrees, and extend to within 1 inch (2.5 cm) of the surface of a firm seat posteriorly. There should be a 2 inch (5.0 cm) gap between the edges of the corset posteriorly. The corset must be worn tight enough to prevent it slipping down over the iliac crests.
— The uprights must be clear of the body, except where pressure is transmitted by pads. The posterior uprights must be perpendicular to the pelvic corset, parallel to each other and pass just medial to the scapulae.
— The neck ring must clear the neck by $\frac{3}{8}$–$\frac{5}{8}$ inches (1.0–1.5 cm) on each side.

— The throat mould must lie $\frac{3}{8}$ inch (1.0 cm) inferior to the mandible and must clear the larynx by a similar distance when the patient's gaze is level.

— The occipital pads must lie inferior to and not behind the occiput, and be bent at an approximate angle of 45 degrees to the vertical.

— Confirm the correct alignment, placement of the pads and the correction of the curve, with antero-posterior radiographs taken in the erect standing position.

Advice to patient and parents

— Advise the patient to wear a cotton vest which is long enough to extend below the pelvic corset. This will protect the skin and keep the brace clean.

— Regular washing and rubbing the skin with alcohol are important. Creams must not be used.

— The brace is worn for 23 hours a day. While wearing the brace the patient must try to lead as normal a life as possible with the exception of contact sports and gymnastics.

— Emphasise to the patient and the parents that the brace is an active corrective spinal brace, and that it is important that the patient carries out exercises twice daily both without the brace and also when wearing it. The patient is instructed in these exercises by a physiotherapist. The exercises are designed to obtain and maintain postural balance, correct the curve, increase muscular strength and improve chest expansion.

— The condition of the patient and the brace is assessed at intervals of three months.

Meralgia paraesthetica can occur during the wearing of a Milwaukee brace (Moe and Kettleson, 1970).

Boston brace (CTLSO) (Fig. 10.9)

The Boston brace* (Hall and Miller, 1974; Asher and Whitney, 1980) is prefabricated from $\frac{1}{8}$ inch (3.0 mm) thick polypropylene. The pelvic corset opens posteriorly. It is vacuum-formed on a positive mould of a normal torso, and is available in twenty different sizes, with the result that approximately 95% of all patients with scoliosis can be fitted. The corset is lined with $\frac{1}{4}$ inch (7.0 mm) thick polyethylene foam with large firmer rolls of foam over the iliac crests.

The brace is designed primarily for the treatment of lumbar and thoraco-lumbar scoliosis in which the apex of the curve is below the eighth thoracic vertebra.

*See Appendix.

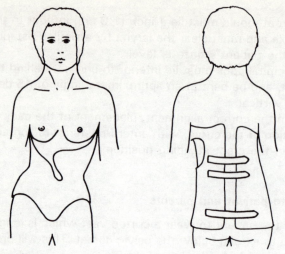

Fig. 10.9 Boston brace.

The checking procedure and advice to the patient and the parents is similar to that for the Milwaukee brace.

ORTHOSES FOR THE CERVICAL SPINE

The head is balanced upon the cervical spine by the action of the neck muscles. The cervical spine exhibits a considerable range of movement in all directions. Inflammatory conditions or mechanical derangements of the cervical spine are associated commonly with spasm of the neck muscles and pain. This spasm and pain may be relieved by heat, massage and exercises, but occasionally immobilization of the cervical spine combined with support of the head to relieve pressure upon the cervical vertebrae, intervertebral discs and joints, and the cervical nerves is required. This can be achieved by spinal traction (see Ch. 6) or by external splintage of the neck.

To immobilize and relieve pressure upon the cervical spine, an external support must be shaped to fit the contours of the lower jaw and occiput, the shoulders, clavicles and sternum and the upper thoracic spine. In the presence of a lesion of the uppermost part of the cervical spine, the forehead also must be included in the support. The inclusion of the thoracic spine and trunk depends upon the level, extent and severity of the lesion of the cervical spine.

For adequate immobilization of a lesion above the level of the sixth thoracic vertebrae, the cervical spine must be immobilized. This is achieved by attaching a cervical support to a long spinal brace, or by prescribing a Milwaukee brace.

There are many different types of cervical orthoses.

Temporary felt or foam collar (CO)
This collar does not control any movement in the cervical spine (Johnson et al, 1977). It consists of a length of orthopaedic felt or foam rubber covered with

stockinette. It is useful in an emergency or when a temporary support is required, for example following muscle strain. It is prepared as follows:

> — Cut a strip of orthopaedic felt or foam rubber measuring 18 inches by 8 inches (45.75 cm by 20.0 cm) and fold it in half lengthways.
> — Cover the felt or foam rubber with stockinette, leaving the ends long, to act as ties.

Thomas's collar (CO)

Many different cervical orthoses are called 'Thomas's Collars'. The original support described by Hugh Owen Thomas was made from sheet metal covered with felt and sheepskin. Thick plastic sheet is used commonly today instead of metal. They (Fig. 10.10) are 'ready-made' and are supplied in different sizes or are adjustable. Great care must be taken to ensure that they are fastened securely around the neck, rest upon the chest and shoulders and support the chin, jaw and occiput. Often they are fitted incorrectly and do not support the cervical spine at all.

Moulded cervical orthoses (CO)

Plastazote. After being heated at 140°C for 5 minutes in a hot-air oven, a piece of Plastazote is moulded around the patient's neck. It is then trimmed and secured with Velcro straps. In this way a support, holding the patient's head in the most comfortable position, can be made accurately and rapidly. Care, however, must be taken while moulding the Plastazote around the neck, especially with men, to allow adequate room for the larynx to move during swallowing.

Polythene. Supports made from polythene (Fig. 10.11) are used usually for immobilization of the cervical spine after operation. However, unlike Plastazote, a plaster model over which the polythene is moulded, must be made first.

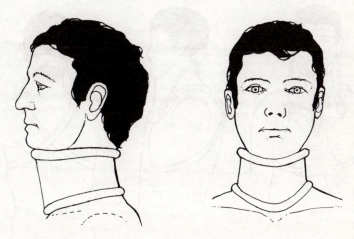

Fig. 10.10 Thomas's collar.

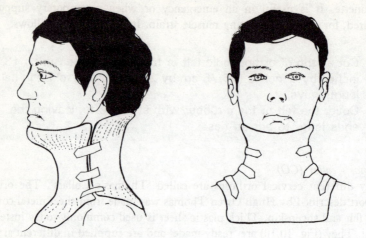

Fig. 10.11 Moulded polythene cervical orthosis.

These cervical orthoses, which have moulded chin and occipital supports, and which extend down over the upper part of the thorax, control flexion and extension between the occiput and the third cervical vertebra (Johnson et al, 1977).

SOMI brace (Fig. 10.12)

The SOMI (Sterno-Occipital-Mandibular-Immobilizer) brace does not have a back plate, and thus allows the patient to lie flat on his back without discomfort. This brace has a padded plastic chest plate and two padded shoulder extensions which hook over the tops of the shoulders. From these shoulder extensions, two straps which cross in the interscapular region, pass downwards and around the chest wall to attach to the lower part of the chest plate. There are three adjustable

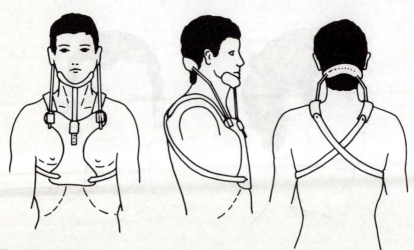

Fig. 10.12 SOMI brace.

uprights which pass upwards from the chest plate, two to the padded occipital support and one to the mandibular support.

This brace can be applied with the patient supine. It is more comfortable than the four-poster cervical brace. It is most effective in controlling foward flexion between the first and fourth cervical vertebrae, especially at the atlanto-axial joint. It is not so effective in controlling extension and lateral flexion (Johnson et al, 1977).

Four-poster cervical brace (Fig. 10.13)
This consists of a padded chin cup and occipital plate attached by four adjustable turnbuckles to two padded plastic plates, one anteriorly and one posteriorly. There are in addition two axillary and two shoulder straps. Two straps connect the chin cup and occipital plate, one on each side of the head.

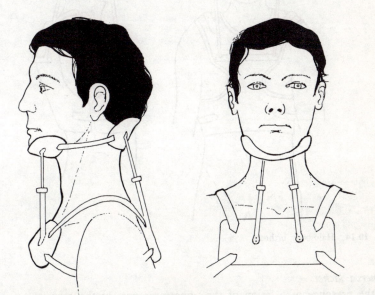

Fig. 10.13 Four-poster cervical brace.

It is easy to apply and adjust. It can be applied prior to radiological examination when bony injury to the cervical spine is suspected.

This brace is effective in limiting flexion in the mid-cervical region, but is less effective in controlling flexion in the lower cervical spine. It does not restrict lateral flexion or rotation (Johnson et al, 1977).

A modification of this brace, in which the chest and back plates extend further down the trunk, and the anterior and posterior components are connected by an encircling thoracic strap with rigid metal connections on each side of the head and over both shoulders, is most effective in controlling flexion and rotation of the lower part, and extension of the upper and middle parts of the cervical spine (Johnson et al, 1977).

Halo-body orthosis* (Fig. 10.14)

The halo-body orthosis and its application are described in detail in Chapter 6. This orthosis consists basically of an oval metal band, the halo, which is fixed to the patient's head just above the eyes and ears, by four metal pins screwed into the outer table of the skull. The halo in turn, is attached to a two-part padded plastic body vest by four adjustable metal uprights, which enables the head to be moved in all directions until the optimum position is obtained.

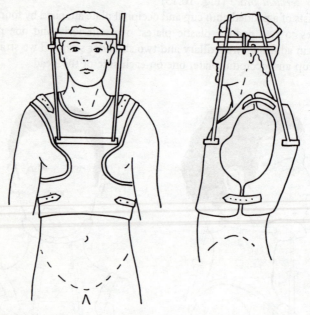

Fig. 10.14 Halo-body orthosis.

Minerva jacket

In the presence of a lesion of the uppermost part of the cervical spine, the forehead also must be included in any external support. As well as the halo-body orthosis, the Minerva jacket, so called because of the similarity of the head portion of the jacket to the shape of a Roman battle helmet, made from plaster-of-Paris, can be used (Fig. 10.15).

PERCENTAGE RESTRICTION OF NORMAL MOVEMENT PROVIDED BY CERVICAL ORTHOSES

The following table is compiled from the findings of Johnson et al (1977) who carried out a study comparing the effectiveness of different cervical orthoses in restricting movement in the cervical spine in normal subjects.

*See Appendix.

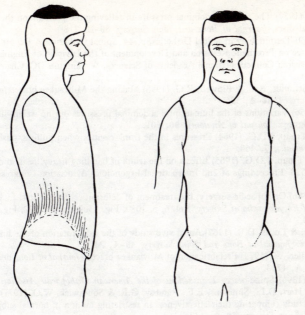

Fig. 10.15 Minerva plaster-of-Paris jacket.

In the following table, the figures represent the percentage reduction in the normal range of movement conferred by the different cervical orthoses.

Table 10.1

	Flexion	Extension	Lat. flexion	Rotation
Soft collar	25	20	10	20
Moulded orthosis	70	60	35	60
Somi brace	95	40	35	70
Four-poster brace	90	80	55	70
Modified four-poster brace	95	90	50	80
Halo-body orthosis	95	95	95	99

It can be seen from this table, that the halo-body orthosis controls movement in the cervical spine better than all the other orthoses. In addition, the way in which the halo is attached to the plastic body vest allows very considerable adjustment of the cervical vertebrae in all directions including longitudinal distraction (see Ch. 6). When accurate control of rotation, lateral flexion and flexion and extension of the cervical spine is required after serious fractures and fracture-dislocations, the halo-body orthosis is the orthosis of choice.

REFERENCES

Allbrook, D. (1957) Movements of the lumbar spinal column. *Journal of Bone and Joint Surgery*, **39–B**, 339.

Asher, M.A. & Whitney, W.H. (1980) Orthotics for spinal deformity. In: Redford, J.B. (ed.) *Orthotics Etcetera*, ch. 7, p. 153, 2nd edn. Baltimore: Williams & Wilkins.

Baker, L.D. (1942) Rhizomelic spondylosis. *Journal of Bone and Joint Surgery*, **24**, 827.

Bartelink, D.L. (1957) The role of abdominal pressure in relieving the pressure on the lumbar intervertebral discs. *Journal of Bone and Joint Surgery,* **39–B,** 718.

Berger, N. (1969) Terminology in Spinal Orthotics, p. 44. Spinal Orthotics: A Report Sponsored by the Committee on Prosthetic Research and Development of the Division of Engineering, National Research Council, National Academy of Sciences, Washington DC, Chairman, H. Elftman.

Blount, W.P., Schmidt, A.C. & Bidwell, R.G. (1958) Making the Milwaukee brace. *Journal of Bone and Joint Surgery,* **40–A,** 526.

Davis, P.R. (1956) Variations of the human intra-abdominal pressures during weight-lifting in different postures. *Journal of Anatomy,* **90,** 601.

Davis, P.R. & Troup, J.D.G. (1964) Pressures in the trunk cavities when pulling, pushing and lifting. *Ergonomics,* **7,** 465.

Davis, P. R. & Troup, J.D.G. (1965) Effects on the trunk of handling heavy loads in different postures p. 323. Proceedings of 2nd International Ergonomics Association Congress. Dortmund 1964.

Fisher, F.R. (1886) Orthopaedic surgery; the treatment of deformities. In Ashurst, J., Jnr (ed.) *International Encyclopaedia of Surgery,* Vol. 6, p. 1080, Fig. 1509 and p. 1082, Fig. 1510. New York: Wood.

Gregersen, G.G. & Lucas, D.B. (1967) An in vivo study of the axial rotation of the human thoraco-lumbar spine. *Journal of Bone and Joint Surgery,* **49–A,** 247.

Hall, J.E. & Miller, W. (1974) Prefabrication of Milwaukee braces. *Journal of Bone and Joint Surgery,* **56–A,** 1763.

Hoadley, A.E. (1896) Spine-brace. *Transactions of the American Orthopaedic Association,* 8, 164.

Johnson, R.M., Hart, D.L., Simmons, E.F., Rambsy, G.R. & Southwick, W.O. (1977) Cervical orthoses: A study comparing their effectiveness in restricting motion in normal subjects. *Journal of Bone and Joint Surgery,* **59–A,** 332.

Jones, R. & Lovett, R.W. (1923) *Orthopaedic Surgery,* p. 236. London: Frowde and Hodder & Stoughton.

Lumsden, R.M. & Morris, J.M. (1968) An in vivo study of axial rotation and immobilisation at the lumbo-sacral joint. *Journal of Bone and Joint Surgery,* **50–A,** 1591.

Moe, J.H. & Kettleson, D.N. (1970) Idiopathic scoliosis. *Journal of Bone and Joint Surgery,* **52–A,** 1509.

Morris, J.M., Lucas, D.B. & Bresler, B. (1961) Role of the trunk in stability of the spine. *Journal of Bone and Joint Surgery,* **43–A,** 327.

Nachemson, A. & Morris, J.M. (1964) In vivo measurements of intra-discal pressure: discometry, a method for the determination of pressure in the lower lumbar discs. *Journal of Bone and Joint Surgery,* **46–A,** 1077.

Nichols, P.J.R., McCay, G. & Bradford, A. (1966) Immediate lumbar supports. *British Medical Journal,* **ii,** 707.

Norton, P.L. & Brown, T. (1957) Immobilising efficiency of back braces: their effect on the posture and motion of the lumbo-sacral spine. *Journal of Bone and Joint Surgery,* **39–A,** 111.

Perry, J. (1970) The use of external support in the treatment of low-back pain. *Journal of Bone and Joint Surgery,* **52–A,** 1440.

Surgical Appliances Contract 1972 (MHM 50), Department of Health and Social Services (D.S.B.4A), Government Buildings, Block 1, Warbreck Hill Road, Blackpool.

Tanz, S.S. (1953) Motion of the lumbar spine: a roentgenologic study. *American Journal of Roentgenology,* **69,** 399.

Taylor, C.F. (1863) On the mechanical treatment of Pott's disease of the spine. *Transactions of the New York State Medical Society,* **6,** 67.

Troup, J.D.G., Hood, C.A. & Chapman, A.E. (1968) Measurements of the sagittal mobility of the lumbar spine and hips. *Annals of Physical Medicine,* **9,** 308.

Van Leuven, R.M. & Troup, J.D.G. (1969) The 'instant' lumbar corset. *Physiotherapy,* **55,** 499.

11.

Lower limb orthoses

A caliper is an orthosis for the lower limb which may be used permanently or for a short time only. Its functions are:

> *To provide stability* for a weakened, paralysed or unstable limb.
> *To relieve weight bearing.*
> *To relieve pain.*
> *To control deformity* aggravated by postural forces.
> *To restrict movement* of the joints of the lower limb.

Two or more of these functions may be combined. The ultimate aim is to enable the patient to walk. To achieve this a caliper must be strong, light and easy to apply and manipulate. In general the more simple an appliance is, the better.

There are two main types of caliper:

WEIGHT-RELIEVING CALIPER (KAFO — Weight Relieving)

The body weight is transmitted from the ischial tuberosity to a padded ring or moulded leather (bucket) top, through metal side bars to the shoe and hence the ground. In practice a weight-relieving caliper provides only partial weight relief. Its use is indicated when it is advisable to decrease the amount of body weight taken through the bones of the lower limb.

CHECKING A WEIGHT-RELIEVING CALIPER

This may be carried out in two ways.
— With the patient supine, lift the splinted leg at right angles to the body. Place the finger between the bearing point of the caliper and the ischial tuberosity. Lower the leg. If the finger is trapped, the length of the caliper is correct. If the finger can easily be removed, the caliper is too short; if the ring slips past the finger, the caliper is too long.

— With the patient standing and sitting back on the caliper top, it should just be possible to slip a finger under the patient's heel.

Advise the patient to sit back on the top of the caliper and to avoid leaning forward with the hip flexed, because as the hip is flexed, the point of contact is transferred forwards progressively from the ischial tuberosity to the ischial ramus and finally the pubic ramus (Young, 1929).

NON WEIGHT-RELIEVING CALIPER (KAFO)

1. Long leg brace (KAFO) similar in design to a weight-relieving caliper but the body weight is *not* supported on a ring. The ring merely locates the upper end of the side bars. This type of caliper is used mainly to control deformity or to restrict the movement of the joints of the lower limb.
2. Below-knee appliance (AFO) used when the ankle or foot alone requires to be controlled.

The basic design of a caliper — two metal side bars connected superiorly by a band encircling the upper thigh, and inferiorly to a shoe — may be modified, depending upon the function required of the caliper. The common variations of each part of a caliper and their functions are described below.

UPPER END OF A CALIPER

The upper end of a caliper may be fitted with a ring, cuff or block leather bucket top.

Ring top

A ring top (Fig. 11.1) consists of a metal ring padded with felt and covered with leather. It may or may not be weight-relieving. If the ring top is to transmit body weight, it must be a snug fit, otherwise the ischial tuberosity will slide through the ring, weight relief will be lost and the ring will press into the perineum where it may cause a pressure sore.

This type of top is often used on calipers for children, or for temporary calipers for adults. It is simple and cheap to construct.

Cuff top

A cuff top (Fig. 11.2) consists of a broad posterior metal thigh band padded with felt and covered with leather. Anteriorly there is a broad soft leather band adjustable by means of a strap and buckle or a Velcro fastening. A cuff top cannot be weight-relieving.

It is simple and cheap to construct, is less bulky than a ring top, and is easy to apply. A cuff top is particularly indicated when, in the presence of marked wasting of the thigh, it would be impossible to pass a ring top of the correct size over the foot or the knee.

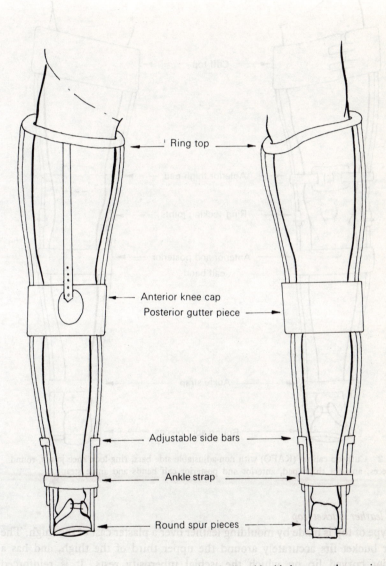

Fig. 11.1 Ring top caliper (KAFO) with unjointed adjustable side bars, round spur pieces, anterior knee cap, posterior gutter piece and ankle strap.

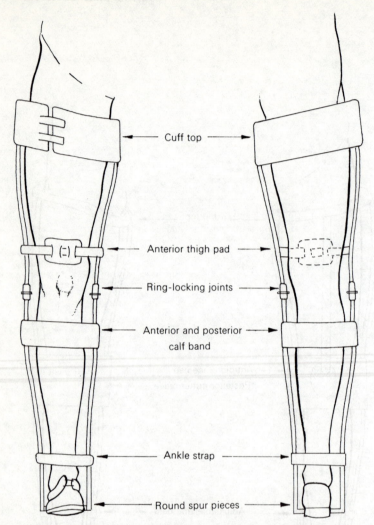

Cuff top

Anterior thigh pad

Ring-locking joints

Anterior and posterior
calf band

Ankle strap

Round spur pieces

Fig. 11.2 Cuff top caliper (KAFO) with non-adjustable side bars, ring-lock knee joints, round spur pieces, anterior thigh pad, anterior and posterior calf bands and ankle strap.

Block leather bucket top

This type of top is made by moulding leather over a plaster cast of the thigh. The leather bucket fits accurately around the upper third of the thigh, and has a posterior curved lip on which the ischial tuberosity rests. It is reinforced posteriorly by a transverse metal band connected to the side bars. A metal strip with a flange projects upwards to support the bucket under the ischial tuberosity. Straps and buckles or lace eyelets are fitted anteriorly (Fig. 11.3).

As this type of top must be made carefully, it is more expensive to manufacture than the other two types. Its use is reserved usually for permanent adult weight-relieving calipers. When the knee is unstable, support can be provided by extending the bucket top downwards to enclose almost the whole thigh.

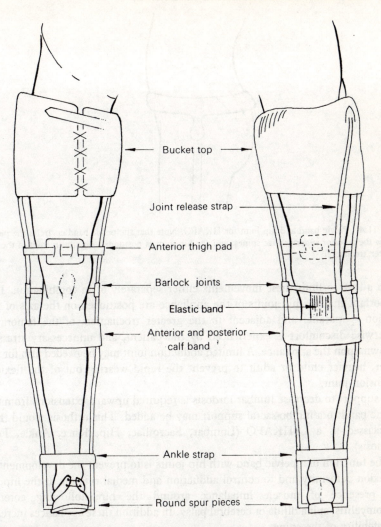

Fig. 11.3 Moulded leather bucket top caliper (KAFO) with non-adjustable side bars, barlock knee joints, round spur pieces, anterior thigh pad, anterior and posterior calf bands and ankle strap.

PELVIC BAND AND HIP JOINTS

A pelvic band is a padded rigid metal band covered with leather which encircles the pelvis posteriorly (extending between the anterior superior iliac spines), and presses on the sacrum. It is fastened anteriorly with a broad padded leather strap and buckle. Lateral metal bands extending downwards from the pelvic band hinge with upward extensions of the lateral side bars of long leg calipers (KAFOs) at the level of the hips (Fig. 11.4). As the orthosis crosses the hip joint it is now called a HKAFO. It is better to use two long leg calipers with a pelvic band. If only one caliper is used, the pelvic band can rotate on the pelvis.

The hinge or hip joint may allow either free flexion or extension, or be fitted

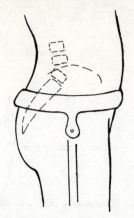

Fig. 11.4 Pelvic band and hip joint for HKAFO. Note that the pelvic band encircles the pelvis below the anterior superior iliac spines, and the hip joint is positioned slightly in front of the greater trochanter.

with a lock to limit these movements either separately or in combination. It is important that the hip joints of the appliance are positioned on the axis of hip flexion — parallel and adjacent to the greater trochanters of the femora — otherwise discomfort is experienced by the patient, and unnecessary stress is thrown upon the appliance. A limited abduction joint may be needed also for the older, heavier child or adult to prevent the rapid wearing out of the flexion-extension joint.

If support to decrease lumbar lordosis is required upward extensions from the pelvic band to a lumbo-sacral support may be added. This orthosis would then be classed as a LSHKAFO (Lumbar, Sacroiliac, Hip, Knee, Ankle, Foot Orthosis).

The function of a pelvic band with hip joints is to prevent the development of a flexion deformity and to control adduction and medial rotation at the hip, in the presence of muscle imbalance around the hip, following anterior poliomyelitis, spina bifida or cerebral palsy. In addition these appliances increase the stability of the spine.

These appliances are always very cumbersome, even although they can be made with only a lateral side bar to the long leg calipers when the pelvic band is well fitting. They should be recommended only after very careful consideration, as the patients who require such appliances are seldom able to walk more than a few yards, even although their stability and mobility may be improved. Light appliances which simply brace the lower limbs may be better, the patient using crutches and a swinging gait.

SIDE BARS

Stability is provided by metal side bars which must be both strong and light. Steel is used for calipers for the lower limbs in heavy patients, the active child, and when severe spasticity or athetosis is present, and for permanent calipers.

Duralumin is suitable for the side bars of light appliances. The moving parts, joints and the attachments of the caliper to the shoe, are always made of steel.

The side bars are shaped to the contour of the limb and must not rub the skin. In children they must be adjustable for length to allow for growth (Fig. 11.1).

The side bars are attached proximally to the ring, cuff or block leather bucket top, and distally are slotted into the heel of the shoe or boot. Knee joints may be incorporated.

KNEE JOINTS

The normal knee is a combination of a hinge and a sliding joint. It is not practicable to make an artificial joint which accurately follows normal knee movement. The nearest point corresponding to the natural axis of movement is situated $\frac{1}{2}$ inch (1.25 cm) above the joint line, and a little posterior to its centre.

Ring lock knee joint
The ring lock knee joint is the safest and most durable. It is illustrated in Figures 11.2 and 11.5. The axis of rotation of the joint is eccentric to prevent the anterior edge of the male section from projecting when the joint is flexed. The ring is pulled up to allow the knee to flex and is pushed downwards when the knee is

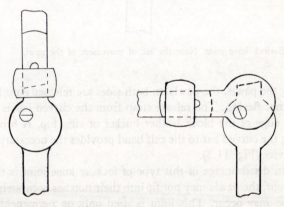

Fig. 11.5 Manual ring-lock knee joint.

extended, to lock the hinge. A spring-loaded ball controls the position of the ring. A patient must have sufficient power in the fingers to manipulate the ring lock. In hemiplegia, the ring lock knee joint must be fitted to the same side of the caliper as the *normal* upper limb, and a simple non-locking joint to the other side bar.

Ring lock knee joints with springs which automatically lock the joint when the knee is extended, may be fitted. An *automatic ring lock* must not be fitted to all four hinges when two calipers are worn, as it is impossible for a patient to manipulate all four ring locks simultaneously while attempting to sit down. A further modification of the automatic ring lock is called the *rod-spring ring lock*.

This consists of a ring lock to the ring of which a length of rod with a co-axial spring is fitted. An upward pull on the rod raises the ring and frees the joint. When the knee is extended, release of the rod allows the co-axial spring to push the ring down and lock the joint. This type of locking knee joint is used when a patient is unable to lean forward far enough to operate an ordinary ring lock knee joint, or when he cannot regain the erect position after bending forward.

Barlock (Swiss lock) knee joint

The barlock type of knee joint (Figs 11.3 and 11.6) locks automatically on extension of the knee. By pulling on a strap attached to a curved posterior bar

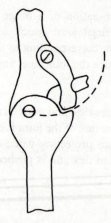

Fig. 11.6 Barlock knee joint. Note the arc of movement of the pawl.

connecting the pawls, the pawls on both sides are released simultaneously, thus allowing knee flexion. The release strap from the curved bar is attached to the top, outer edge of the block leather bucket or ring top. A broad elastic band connecting the curved bar to the calf band provides the necessary tension for the locking device (Fig. 11.3).

The main disadvantage of this type of locking knee joint is that with lateral malalignment, the pawls may not fit into their notches accurately, and therefore malfunction may occur. This joint is used only on permanent appliances for patients who will always have to walk with an extended knee, as this joint cannot be left unlocked. The barlock knee joint must never be used when spasticity is present, as failure is very likely to occur.

It is important that this type of knee joint is manufactured correctly. The tips of the pawls move through an arc of a circle. To ensure accurate locking, the lugs on the distal side of the knee joint must lie on the same arc, and must therefore point upwards and backwards (Fig. 11.6).

Posterior off-set knee joint (Fig. 11.7)

The posterior off-set knee joint is a non-locking type of joint. When incorporated into a long leg caliper, the axis of movement of the joint is situated posterior to the axis of flexion/extension of the knee. This means that when the knee is in at

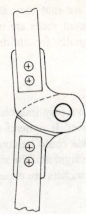

Fig. 11.7 Posterior off-set knee joint.

least 10 degrees of hyperextension, the posterior off-set knee joint is stable as the body weight passes down a line anterior to the axis of movement of the joint.

These types of knee joints are used instead of locking knee joints in the 'cosmetic' appliances, which have been introduced recently, for patients with a flail lower limb who exhibit at least 10 degrees of hyperextension at the knee (see later). Hyperextension can be aided if necessary by lowering the heel of the shoe slightly and adding a small raise to the sole.

Knee joints usually are not fitted to children's calipers. Locking knee joints may be essential for a spastic child or to aid in sitting at school. They are reserved for permanent adult calipers, either weight relieving or non-weight relieving, to ease sitting.

HEEL ATTACHMENT OF SIDE BARS

The distal ends of a caliper may be attached to the shoe or boot by means of heel sockets or via a stirrup.

HEEL SOCKETS

The distal ends of the side bars of a caliper are bent inwards at a right angle and slotted into metal sockets fitted into the heel of the shoe. The caliper ends (spur pieces) and the heel sockets may be round or flat (rectangular).

Round sockets
These are employed when muscle control is adequate and the patient is able to dorsiflex and plantar-flex his ankle. The disadvantages of the round socket are that movement at the anatomical ankle joint does not correspond with the level of the ankle joint of the appliance, with the result that the appliance rides up and down with dorsiflexion and plantar-flexion; compression of the calf by the calf band occurs on dorsiflexion; and the heel tends to slip out of the shoe. The

advantages of round sockets are that they are easier to make and adjust, the apparatus is lighter, and different shoes are interchangeable easily.

Round sockets are used usually for children's calipers, and for temporary calipers for adults.

Flat (or rectangular) sockets

This type of heel socket allows easy interchangeability of shoes but does not allow the heel of the shoe to pivot. It is therefore usually employed with an ankle hinge (Fig. 11.12). A flail ankle could be controlled by flat sockets without an ankle hinge, but fixation is too rigid and the shoe would not withstand the strain unless it was reinforced. Flat sockets are expensive and are reserved usually for permanent calipers.

STIRRUPS

There are two types of stirrup attachment, the ordinary stirrup and the sandal or insert stirrup.

Ordinary stirrup

An ordinary stirrup consists of a U-shaped piece of metal which is rigidly fixed to the anterior part of the underside of the heel of the shoe. The arms of the U pass up and slightly backwards (about 5–6 degrees) on each side of the shoe to ankle joints positioned on the axis of movement of the anatomical ankle joint.

Sandal or insert type of stirrup

In this type a footplate is attached to the stirrup, both of which are placed inside the shoe (Fig. 11.8). The main advantage of this method is that shoes can be changed easily. Moreover, as the foot plate and stirrup take up room in the shoe, it may be possible to wear shoes of the same size when there is a discrepancy in the size of the feet, as may occur in patients who have had poliomyelitis. The disadvantages of the sandal type of stirrup are that pressure sores may develop,

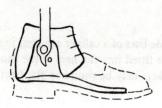

Fig. 11.8 Sandal or insert type of stirrup.

and control of movement between the foot and the foot plate is difficult. The sandal type of stirrup must never be used for patients with paraplegia or sensory disturbance in the foot.

TOE-OUT

When arranging the attachment of the side bars of a caliper to a shoe by any of the above methods, it is necessary to provide toe-out, to prevent the patient from tripping over his toes. The amount of toe-out required is determined individually. It depends upon the relationship between the axes of movement of the knee and ankle joints, which in turn depends upon the degree of tibial torsion present. The amount of toe-out usually provided is 10 to 15 degrees. To achieve this the attachment of the inner side bar of the caliper is positioned slightly posterior to that of the outer side bar (Fig. 11.9).

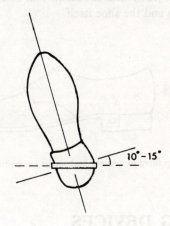

Fig. 11.9   Toe-out.

ANKLE JOINTS

A joint at the level of the ankle follows the natural ankle movement. It can be constructed to allow free movement, or to limit plantar-flexion or dorsiflexion or both.

It is essential that the axes of movement of the mechanical and anatomical ankle joints are identical. The axis of anatomical movement lies on a line which passes from just below the tip of the medial malleolus and which bisects the lateral malleolus one half inch above its tip.

When ankle joints are incorporated in a caliper, flat heel sockets (Fig. 11.12) or a stirrup are necessary. As these fittings are difficult and expensive to make, they are reserved usually for permanent adult calipers or when a toe raising device is required.

CONTROL OF ANKLE JOINT MOVEMENT (AFO)

Movement at the anatomical ankle joint can be controlled by specially constructed mechanical ankle joints, or, when round heel sockets are used, by heel stops.

Heel stop

This is a metal lug attached to the anterior or posterior aspects of a round heel socket (Fig. 11.10), to limit dorsiflexion or plantar-flexion respectively. If plantar-flexion is weak, excessive dorsiflexion can be controlled with a front or calcaneus stop. Conversely if dorsiflexion is weak, foot control can be improved by adding a back or equinus stop. In the presence of a flail ankle, front and back stops can be fitted so that only a few degrees of dorsiflexion and plantar-flexion are possible. The main disadvantage of this method of controlling ankle movement is that the axis of movement of the appliance does not correspond with that of the ankle joint, with the result that considerable stress is imposed upon the heel sockets and the shoe itself.

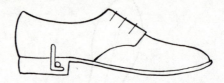

Fig. 11.10 Back heel stop fitted to a round heel socket to control plantar-flexion at the ankle joint (AFO–Plantar S).

TOE-RAISING DEVICES

When weakness of dorsiflexion is present, the fitting of a device to aid dorsiflexion will improve greatly the patient's function. Tripping over uneven ground and the characteristic high stepping gait will be abolished. As stated above, the fitting of a back stop or a mechanical ankle joint constructed to control plantar-flexion will passively control a drop foot. There are however a number of active methods employed which utilise a spring device of some sort.

Double below-knee iron, round heel sockets and toe-raising spring (AFO Dorsi A: Ankle, Foot Orthosis   Dorsiflexion Assist)
The simplest type of toe-raising spring is illustrated in Figure 11.11. The spring is attached to the double below-knee iron which fits into round heel sockets, by a Y-shaped strap. The lower end of the spring is attached to the middle of the dorsum of the shoe, at the level of the metatarso-phalangeal joints, by a small leather lug stitched to the shoe. This is a cheap and effective mechanism but it is obvious, especially when worn by women, and considerable stress is imposed upon the heel sockets and the shoe.

Double below-knee iron, ankle joints, flat heel sockets and toe-raising spring (AFO
    Dorsi A: Ankle, Foot Orthosis   Dorsiflexion Assist)
A less obvious toe-raising spring is that employed with an ankle joint and flat spur pieces and heel sockets as illustrated in Figure 11.12. The spring is attached

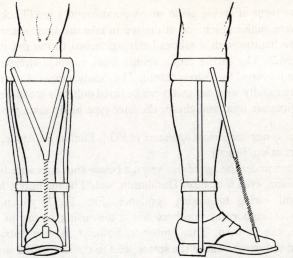

Fig. 11.11 Double below-knee iron, round spur pieces, toe-raising spring and ankle strap (AFO–Dorsi A).

to the outer side bar (or both side bars) of a caliper or double below-knee iron by an adjustable strap and buckle or wire rod, and to a lug projecting forward from the centre of the ankle joint. This apparatus is heavy and expensive. Considerable stress is still imposed upon the shoe and heel sockets, and with time the flat spur pieces become worn and loose.

Double below-knee iron with rubber torsion socket (AFO   Plantar R: Ankle, Foot Orthosis   Plantarflexion Resist)
When the force required to overcome the drop foot is not great, a toe-raising device concealed in the heel can be used. Originally this device consisted of a

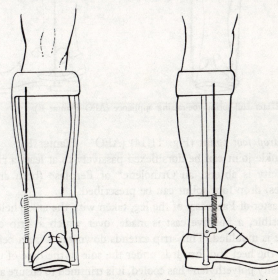

Fig. 11.12 Double below-knee iron with ankle joints, flat spur pieces, toe-raising spring and ankle strap (AFO–Dorsi A).

number of turns of spring piano wire wound round a rod (Tuck, 1957). Square sockets were sunk in each end of the rod to take the spur pieces. A similar toe-raising mechanism with a rubber bush vulcanised to the rod is now available (Tuck, 1962). The spring action results from torsional stresses in the rubber which can be varied by a screw thread. The disadvantages of the rubber bush are that it may rapidly wear out and it can be fitted only to a broad-heeled shoe. Both these devices are light and cheap, the later type being mass produced.

Exeter coil spring toe-raising appliance (AFO   Plantar R: Ankle, Foot Orthosis Plantarflexion Resist)

For children under the age of five years, a below-knee appliance fitted with a toe-raising spring, even if made of Duralumin, would be too heavy. In such cases an Exeter coil spring toe-raising appliance (Fig. 11.13) which combines the functions of supporting side bars and a toe-raising spring in a simple light appliance, can be used. This appliance, however, is very restrictive, with the result that the attachment of the spring steel to the heel of the shoe may become loose, or the steel itself may break.

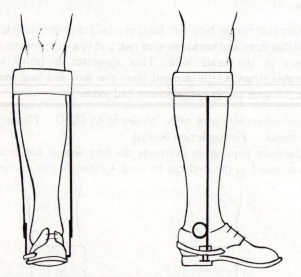

Fig. 11.13   Exeter coil-spring toe-raising appliance (AFO–Plantar R).

Ortholene★ drop foot splint (Fig. 11.14) (AFO   Plantar R)

When the ankle joint can be dorsiflexed passively to at least a right angle, and when spasticity is absent, an Ortholene★ or Perplas★ (both are high-density polyethylenes) drop foot splint can be prescribed.

From a plaster-of-Paris cast of the leg, taken with the ankle held above a right angle if possible, a positive cast is made, over which a strip of high-density polyethylene is moulded. This strip extends downwards from behind the upper calf, around the heel and forwards under the sole to the base of the toes. When the high-density polyethylene has cooled, it is trimmed to ensure a snug fit inside

★See Appendix.

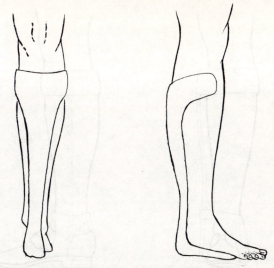

Fig. 11.14 Ortholene drop foot splint (AFO–Plantar R).

the shoe, and the edges are chamfered, especially under the toes. If necessary a calf pad of Plastazote can be added to improve the cosmetic appearance of the leg.

The splint is worn next to the skin. A Velcro strap may be fitted to the upper end to keep it closely applied to the back of the calf, or an elastic stocking may be worn.

This splint overcomes the cosmetic and mechanical disadvantages of the previously described appliances. In addition it overcomes the disadvantage of some of the present-day commercial footwear, the heels of which are hollow plastic mouldings unsuitable for the insertion of heel sockets.

T-STRAPS

A T-strap is cut from leather. The vertical limb of the T is attached to the shoe at the junction of the upper with the sole. It is placed well forward. The strap is cut with long tongues so that the upper end of the strap encircles both the ankle and the side bar with the buckle on the other side of the leg, and the end of the strap pointing backwards.

A T-strap may be attached to either the inside or the outside of the shoe, to provide stability and to substitute for paralysed or partially paralysed invertor or evertor muscles. A single below-knee appliance (side bar) is used in conjunction with a T-strap (Fig. 11.15).

Examples:

1. When the tibialis anterior and tibialis posterior muscles are weak, but the peroneal muscles are strong, the foot will assume a position of valgus. This deformity can be controlled by an outside iron and an inside T-strap.

2. A varus deformity from weakness of the peroneal muscles can be controlled with an inside iron and an outside T-strap.

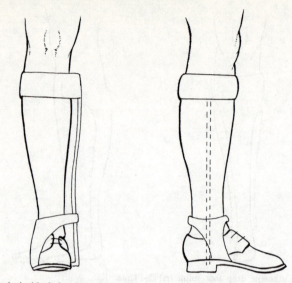

Fig. 11.15 Single inside below-knee iron with round spur piece and outside T-strap (AFO).

RETAINING STRAPS AND BANDS

In addition to the above modifications which may be made to a caliper, it must be remembered that the limb must be retained within the caliper. This is achieved by using various leather straps and bands. These are described below.

Ankle strap
The spur pieces of an appliance must be retained in the heel sockets. A T-strap will perform this function as well as correcting a varus or valgus deformity. In the absence of a T-strap, an ankle strap must be present. An ankle strap is attached to the outer side bar, passes around the inner side bar and lower part of the leg, and back to the outer side bar where it is buckled firmly (Figs 11.1, 11.2, 11.3, 11.11, 11.12, 11.17).

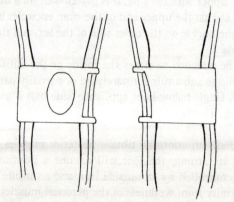

Fig. 11.16 Knock-knee pad.

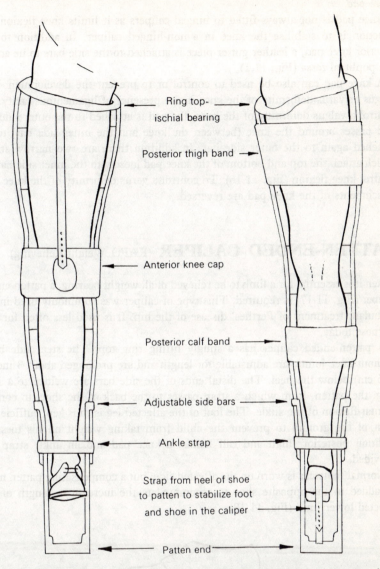

Ring top-
ischial bearing

Posterior thigh band

Anterior knee cap

Posterior calf band

Adjustable side bars

Ankle strap

Strap from heel of shoe
to patten to stabilize foot
and shoe in the caliper

Patten end

Fig. 11.17 Patten ended caliper (KAFO–Weight relieving) with ischial bearing ring top, adjustable side bars, posterior thigh band, anterior knee cap, posterior calf band, ankle strap and strap from heel of shoe to patten.

Calf band and anterior thigh pad
When a knee joint is used a calf band and an anterior thigh pad are fitted. The calf band, lined with felt and covered with leather, is attached to the side bars just below the knee joint. A padded anterior thigh pad is fitted above the knee joint (Figs 11.2, 11.3). It is not required when a long leather bucket top is used. The calf band and the anterior thigh pad are fastened with a strap and buckle or a Velcro fastening. Eyelets and a lace can also be used for the latter.

Knee pad

A knee pad is not always fitted to hinged calipers as it limits knee flexion. Its function is to stabilise the knee in a non-hinged caliper. In addition to the anterior knee pad, a leather gutter piece is attached to the side bars to lie across the popliteal fossa (Fig. 11.1).

A knee pad can also be used to control or to prevent the development of a valgus or varus deformity of the knee in the presence of ligamentous laxity. To control a valgus deformity of the knee, the pad is attached to the outer side bar and passes around the knee (between the knee and the inner side bar) to be attached again to the outer side bar. In addition there are two narrow straps which attach the top and bottom of the knee pad loosely to the inner side bar, to control knee flexion (Fig. 11.16). To control a varus deformity of the knee, the attachments of the knee pad are reversed.

PATTEN-ENDED CALIPER (KAFO Weight-Relieving)

When it is essential for a limb to be relieved of all weight bearing, a patten-ended caliper (Fig. 11.17) is required. This type of caliper was commonly used in the ambulant treatment of Perthes' disease of the hip. It is used less often for this purpose today.

A patten-ended caliper has a snugly fitting ring top. The steel side bars, without knee joints, are adjustable for length and are prolonged about 3 inches (7.6 cm) below the heel. The distal ends of the side bars are welded to a steel ring, the patten, from which a strap passes to the back of the shoe, to control plantar-flexion of the ankle. The foot of the affected leg is thus kept sufficiently clear of the ground to prevent the child from taking weight on his toes. In addition posterior thigh and calf bands, a knee pad and an ankle strap are provided.

Normal footwear is worn on the affected side, but a compensating patten must be added to the opposite shoe to accommodate the increase in length of the affected lower limb (Fig. 11.18).

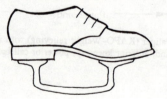

Fig. 11.18 Compensatory patten on a normal shoe.

The length of the caliper must be adjusted repeatedly to allow for growth, otherwise the child will soon bear weight on its toes. Whether or not this is occurring can be determined by examining the toe of the shoe worn on the affected side, for the presence of wear.

THE 'COSMETIC' LONG LEG CALIPER (KAFO)
(Fig. 11.19)

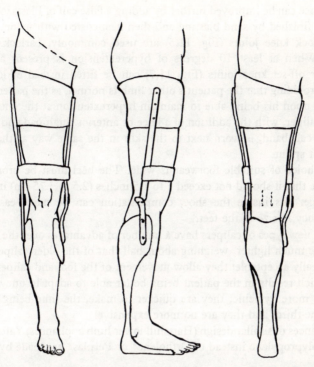

Fig. 11.19 'Cosmetic' long leg caliper (KAFO). Note that the side bars end just below the knee where they are riveted to an Ortholene drop foot splint. Posterior off-set knee joints are illustrated.

The long leg calipers illustrated in Figures 11.1, 11.2 and 11.3 have a number of disadvantages. They are cumbersome, heavy, rigid and often uncomfortable. They frequently break, are not cosmetically acceptable especially to women, and take many hours to make. In addition all the patient's shoes have to be fitted with heel sockets, and as the foot of the affected limb is often smaller, the patient may have to buy two pairs of shoes each time.

To overcome these inherent disadvantages and the additional problem of the unsuitable present-day commercial footwear, a new type of non-weight relieving long leg caliper (KAFO) for use in cases of flaccid paralysis of the lower limb has been developed by Mr W.H. Tuck at The Royal National Orthopaedic Hospital. This development has resulted from the introduction of plastics and has received additional impetus from the previous development of the Ortholene drop foot splint.

This new appliance is fitted with a bucket top made from high-density polyethylene moulded around a positive cast of the upper thigh and ischial region. Where the shape and size of the foot will allow, the bucket top is riveted, forming a rigid cylinder which is threaded over the limb when the caliper is applied.

The side bars terminate just below the knee where they are riveted to a modified Ortholene drop foot splint. This results in the caliper being lighter, and more resilient and cosmetically acceptable to the patient. The cosmetic appearance can be improved further by adding a false calf of Plastazote. The side bars are finished by sand blasting and then heat-coated with nylon.

Ring-lock knee joints (Fig. 11.5) are used commonly, barlock joints only rarely. When at least 10 degrees of hyperextension is present at the knee, posterior off-set knee joints (Fig. 11.7) can be fitted instead of locking knee joints, providing that the patient's other limb is normal, as the patient's stability depends upon his being able to maintain hyperextension at the knee.

The caliper, with the addition of a knee or anterior thigh pad and possibly an anterior calf band, is worn next to the skin in the same way as the Ortholene drop-foot splint.

The choice of suitable footwear is wide. The heel must be broad and it is advisable that it should not exceed 1 to 1.5 inches (2.5 to 3.75 cm) in height. As the caliper fits inside the shoe, compensation can be made easily for any discrepancy in size of the feet.

These new types of calipers have a number of advantages over the older types. They are much lighter, weighing about half that of the older calipers; they are cosmetically acceptable; they allow movement of the foot and caliper within the shoe which results in the patient being better able to adapt to uneven surfaces; they are more hygienic; they are quicker to make, the time being reduced by about one-third; and they are no more expensive.

Appliances of similar design (Hartshill lower limb appliances, Yates, 1968) but using polypropylene instead of Ortholene* or Perplas* are made by Salt & Son Ltd.*

PRESCRIPTION, CHECKING AND CARE OF CALIPERS

The prescription, checking and care of calipers is considered in Chapter 9.

REFERENCES

Tuck W.H. (1957) Drop-foot appliance with concealed spring. *Journal of Bone and Joint Surgery*, **39–B,** 335.
Tuck, W.H. (1962) Drop-foot appliance with rubber torsion socket. *Journal of Bone and Joint Surgery*, **44–B,** 896.
Yates, G. (1968) A method for the provision of lightweight aesthetic orthopaedic appliances. *Orthopaedics*, Oxford, **1,** 153.
Young, C.S. (1929) A study in fitting the ring of the Thomas splint. *Journal of the American Medical Association*, **93,** 602.

*See Appendix.

12.

Footwear

The most important requirement of any footwear is that it fits correctly. If footwear fits correctly, it will be comfortable and will not cause pain or deformity in the future.

Any attempt to accommodate normal feet within incorrect footwear will result in pain, the formation of callosities, bursae and skin ulceration from localised areas of excessive pressure, and occasionally, growth abnormalities. If the feet are deformed, the above complications are more likely to occur.

The shape of a normal foot is not symmetrical. It changes with growth in childhood, in length more rapidly than in width, as well as with age and increasing weight in adult life. The foot increases in length and width on standing, and one foot may be larger than the other.

Many people, women more than men, do not wear suitable footwear and do not understand why their feet are painful. It is important therefore to examine carefully the footwear of all patients complaining of painful feet. When this is done, it is often obvious that their footwear does not fit correctly, and that their feet are being squeezed. Some women are slaves to fashion, and will persist in wearing so-called fashionable shoes which they feel make them look more attractive. In addition, they frequently insist on buying a size 6B for example, because that it is the size they have always bought, and wearing footwear with high heels which tends to push the foot forward, cramping the toes and thus predisposing to the development of deformities of the toes and metatarsalgia.

There are a number of different factors which contribute to the problem of obtaining suitable footwear, even for normal feet, such as:

1. The confusion in sizes between footwear made in different countries.
2. Some styles of footwear are only available in one or certainly a limited number of widths.
3. The shape of the shoe or boot itself.
4. The lack of adequately trained staff in shoeshops to advise customers on suitable footwear.
5. The psychological barrier, especially with women, to accepting that the size of their feet may change with age.

6. The lack of education in the problems which can result from incorrect and ill-fitting footwear.
7. The failure to have *both* feet measured for length and width *while standing*, every time new footwear is purchased.

THE NORMAL SHOE

To enable a doctor to communicate with an orthotist, a basic understanding of the construction of footwear is essential.

A shoe is built over a last which is a model of the weight-bearing foot. The main parts of a shoe are the upper, the sole, the heel, the linings and the reinforcements.

THE UPPER

The upper is that part of the shoe above the sole (Fig. 12.1). It is divided into an anterior part, the vamp, and a posterior part, the quarters, medial and lateral. The lateral quarter must be cut low enough to avoid pressure on the lateral malleolus.

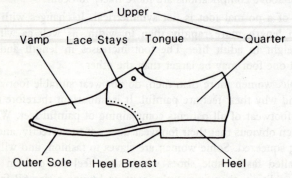

Fig. 12.1 The main parts of a normal shoe.

Eyelets for the laces are situated in the lace stays under which lies the tongue. At the base of the tongue is the throat of the shoe, through which the foot enters. The lace stays may or may not be a part of the vamp, depending upon the style of the shoe.

In the *Gibson* style of shoe (Fig. 12.2), the quarters are stitched on top of the vamp so that the lace stays open freely to allow the foot to enter. A comparable style of boot is termed *Derby*.

In the *Oxford* style of shoe (Fig. 12.3), the vamp overlies the quarters which meet at the front and are laced together. *Balmoral* is the term given to a boot of similar style. The Oxford style does not allow the tongue of the shoe to be reflected back as far as in the Gibson style, as a result the shoe cannot be opened as widely to allow the foot to enter the shoe.

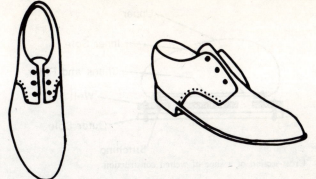

Fig. 12.2 The Gibson style of shoe. Note the plain vamp.

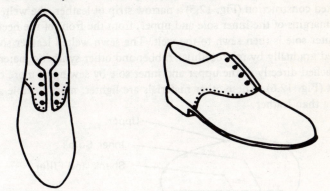

Fig. 12.3 The Oxford style of shoe. Note that the vamp overlies the quarters thus limiting how wide the shoe can be opened to allow the foot to enter.

THE SOLE

There are two soles. The outer sole is separated from the inner sole on which the foot rests, by a compressible filler and the shank. The shank is a rigid strip of steel, extending from the middle of the heel forwards to $\frac{1}{4}-\frac{3}{8}$ inches (6.0–9.0 mm) behind the break of the shoe which corresponds to the line of the metatarsophalangeal joints. The shank reinforces the waist of the shoe, which is that part of the shoe which lies between the heel breast (see below) and the broadest part of the sole, the ball (Fig. 12.4).

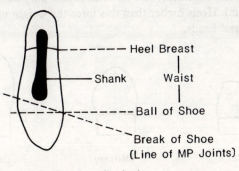

Fig. 12.4 The outer sole is reinforced by the shank.

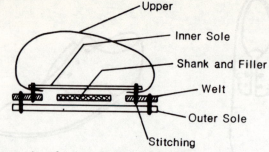

Fig. 12.5 Cross-section of a shoe of welted construction.

The outer sole can be attached in two ways — indirectly or welted, or directly. In welted construction (Fig. 12.5) a narrow strip of leather, the welt, is stitched to the margins of the inner sole and upper, from the front of the heel forwards. The outer sole is then sewn to the welt. The sewn welted leather sole is being replaced gradually by microcellular rubber and other synthetic materials which are attached directly to the upper and inner sole by sewing or more commonly, cement (Fig. 12.6). These other materials are lighter, more flexible and harder wearing than leather.

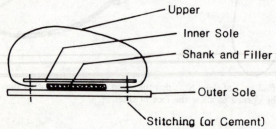

Fig. 12.6 Cross-section of a shoe where the sole is attached directly to the upper and inner sole either by stitching or cement.

THE HEEL

The anterior surface of the heel is called the heel breast (Figs 12.1, 12.4). The shape of the heel may vary (Fig. 12.7). It should have straight sides and be broad enough, unlike the stilleto heel, to provide firm support and prevent the ankle from rolling over. The height is measured in front of the centre of the heel, in line with the medial malleolus, and for orthopaedic purposes should not exceed $1\frac{5}{8}$ inches (4.2 cm). Heels higher than this force the weight of the body forward onto the metatarsal heads.

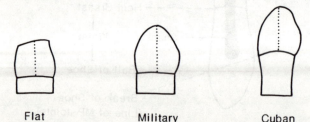

Flat   Military   Cuban

Fig. 12.7 Different types of heel. For orthopaedic purposes the height of the heel should not exceed $1\frac{5}{8}$ inches (4.2 cm).

THE LININGS

Those parts of the shoe which make contact with the foot are lined. The vamp is lined with cotton and the inner sole and the quarters with either leather, or cotton reinforced with leather.

REINFORCEMENTS

The vamp is reinforced by the toe box, and the quarters, in the area of the anatomical heel, by the counters (Fig. 12.8).

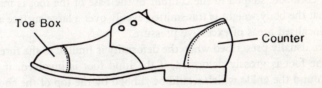

Toe Box

Counter

Fig. 12.8 The toe box and counter which reinforce the toe and the back of the shoe in the region of the anatomical heel, respectively.

SURGICAL FOOTWEAR

The manufacture of special footwear, or alterations or additions to existing footwear, may be necessary to accommodate deformed feet, to relieve pain, to compensate for shortening of a lower limb, or to provide the foundation for an orthosis. When doubt exists as to what is best to relieve a patient's symptoms, consult the orthotist.

The provision of well-fitting individually made surgical footwear is becoming more and more difficult as fewer people are being trained in this skilled work (Shaw, 1976). Unfortunately as the range of footwear available in the usual commercial field becomes more limited, there has been an increase in the demand for surgical footwear, thus compounding the problem.

The comfort of the patient is paramount. It is sometimes possible to fulfil this aim without prescribing surgical footwear. Giving the patient advice about suitable footwear may be all that is necessary. Other patients can be referred to a local shop which may stock a larger range of sizes, be given the address of firms which supply footwear in extra wide fittings (Bury Boot and Shoe Co. Ltd*), or be supplied with stock shoes of greater depth than normal, to allow more room for deformed toes, or to accept insoles. Others may only require modifications to their normal footwear.

The supply of individually made surgical footwear is best supervised by one person, from the taking of measurements or a cast of the foot, through making the last and shoe, to fitting and final supply. In Great Britain, much of the

---

*See Appendix.

present surgical footwear is made in factories many miles away from the patient by someone who has never seen the patient's foot. This difficulty also existed in the United States of America but has been overcome by the Veterans Administration with the development of their orthopaedic shoe service (Staros, 1976).

Surgical footwear is made on a last constructed from accurate measurements or from a plaster cast of the deformed foot.

When a foot is deformed, for example by hammer toes or hallux valgus, but is still plantigrade, careful measurements of the foot are adequate for the construction of the last. When the abnormality of the foot is such that the plantar surface of the foot cannot be accommodated on a leather sole, for example severe untreated talipes equino-varus, a preliminary plaster cast of the foot is essential. An inside cork sole shaped to the contour of the base of the foot is made. This ensures that the body weight is transmitted evenly over a large surface area, thus avoiding localised areas of excessive pressure.

Shoes are usually prescribed when the deformity is limited to the forefoot, and boots if the foot is grossly deformed, if the hind foot is involved, if scars are present around the ankle which would be rubbed by the top of the shoe, or if a large raise is required.

Boots grip the feet better than shoes, reducing piston action, and thus resisting the tendency of the feet to slide backwards and forwards.

The vamp of surgical shoes and boots is commonly plain, as this gives a smooth inner surface.

When surgical footwear is prescribed, consideration must also be given to the size of the opening through which the foot is to be inserted. The Oxford style cannot be opened widely over the forefoot, whereas the Gibson style can be, thus easing the insertion of a more rigid foot into the shoe. A very rigid or flail foot requires an even larger opening. This is provided by lacing extending distally to the toes (Fig. 12.9). Piedro* and Eagle* lace-to-toe bootees are suitable for supply to children and some adults with small feet, suffering from spina bifida and other conditions with gross neurological disorders of the feet.

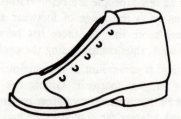

Fig. 12.9 Boot with lacing extending distally to the toes thus allowing a much wider opening for entry of the foot. Note that the eyelets have been replaced with hooks.

It is important also to consider the method of closure of the shoe or boot. The most common method of closure by laces and eyelets allows the snugness of the vamp to be adjusted to accommodate swelling of the feet. On boots, some or all of the eyelets may be replaced by hooks, thus enabling the patient to don and doff the boots more rapidly, especially if hand function is impaired. Some patients

*See Appendix.

with impaired hand function, or limitation of elbow, knee or hip movement may not be able to manage normal laces. The replacement of ordinary laces with elastic laces (Soesi laces*) or the use of footwear of the slip-on variety, can be of great help in such situations. Elastic shoe laces are not suitable for use with an ankle-foot orthosis. Strap and buckle, and Velcro flaps afford other methods of easily adjustable closure. The Velcro flaps can be sewn on over the lace stays. Shoes or boots may be fitted with Zip-fasteners or elastic webbing inserts; with neither can the snugness of fit be adjusted. Sometimes a long-handled shoe horn can be of great benefit.

Vacuum-formed Plastazote and Yampi footwear (Tuck, 1971)
Over the last few years many new synthetic materials have been developed. These are now beginning to be used in the manufacture of surgical footwear. From materials such as Plastazote* (a high-density polyethylene) covered with Yampi* (a plastic), vacuum-formed shoes and bootees can be made.

This type of footwear may be used in the conservative management of any severely deformed foot, such as may occur in rheumatoid arthritis, after partial amputation or leprosy, or when trophic ulceration or gross swelling is present. Shoes or bootees can be made, the latter being prescribed when the foot is severely deformed.

A preliminary plaster-of-Paris cast of the foot is taken, from which a positive plaster cast is made. A Plastazote inner sole is initially formed, and is then added to and trimmed as necessary to obtain a flat surface. The upper is then formed, and after trimming it is attached to the inner sole with an adhesive. A microcellular sole and heel and a Velcro fixing are added finally.

This type of footwear has a number of advantages over the presently accepted surgical shoes and boots. It fits snugly around the heel and mid-foot; it provides total surface contact with the sole of the foot, thus ensuring that the body-weight is spread evenly over a large area and that localised areas of excessive pressure are avoided; it is about one-third the weight of similar leather footwear; it can be washed and is therefore more hygienic; the Velcro fixing is managed easily even by severely deformed hands; and it will last for up to twelve months. The main disadvantages are that some patients experience excessive sweating of their feet and the appearance is not so smart as that of leather footwear.

This type of footwear is available commercially in a range of stock sizes (Drushoe*; Dermaplast*).

The Drushoes (Fig. 12.10) do not have any seams except at the heel. They are

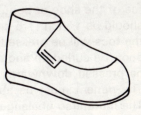

 Standard Depth    Extra Depth

Fig. 12.10 Drushoes, of standard depth on the left and of extra-depth on the right.

*See Appendix.

supplied with two removable insoles, in eleven sizes, two colours (black and brown) and in two forms (standard and extra-depth). The Drushoe may be worn as supplied, cut down to form a shoe or sandal (Fig. 12.11), or be moulded to the patient's foot after locally heating with a hair dryer, or after heating in a hot air oven for two minutes at 140°C. The sole of the Drushoe is adequate for outdoor use.

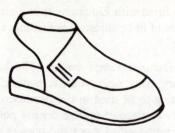

Fig. 12.11 Drushoe where the quarters have been removed.

HOW TO CHECK THAT FOOTWEAR FITS CORRECTLY

The fit of any footwear is of the greatest importance during weight bearing and walking because of the tendency for the foot to lengthen and become broader, due to the stretching of the ligaments of the foot, under the influence of body weight. Therefore the patient must be asked to stand and walk when footwear is checked.

— Excessive pressure must not be exerted on the foot by the upper or the inner sole.

— The fit must be snug enough so that the shoe does not fall off the foot, but loose enough for movement of the foot to occur within the shoe with walking and running.

— There must be adequate clearance over the dorsum of the toes, as well as adequate space at the sides of the heads of the first and fifth metatarsal heads. If the shoe is not deep or wide enough, the metatarsal heads will be pressed downwards.

— There must be a gap between the ends of all the toes and the toe of the shoe or boot. With respect to the hallux this gap should be $\frac{5}{8}$ inch (1.5 cm). If the shoe or boot is too short, the toes will be pressed against the inside of the shoe or boot, be curled up and again cause the metatarsal heads to be pressed downwards.

— The patient must be able to move all his toes freely.

— The metatarso-phalangeal joint of the hallux must be level with the inner curve of the sole, where the sole starts to curve laterally under the arch.

— The counters must fit snugly around the back of the patient's heel.
— The quarters must not gape excessively.
— The quarters must not rub on the malleoli.
— The waist of the shoe or boot must grip the foot firmly enough to prevent the foot from slipping forward or backward.
— The quarters must be high enough medially over the instep to prevent impingement or irritation at or near the region of the first metatarso-medial cuneiform joint. If it is not high enough in this region, then if the laces are tied tightly, there will be a tendency for the medial arch to be pushed downwards, elongating the foot.

MODIFICATIONS TO EXISTING FOOTWEAR

Although surgical footwear, as discussed above, may be required for the management of painful feet, particularly in the case of severe deformity, much foot pain can be alleviated by prescribing various additions or alterations to existing footwear. An accurate diagnosis must be made before these additions or alterations are prescribed. It must be remembered that often foot symptoms can be relieved by physiotherapy.

Some modern shoes are not suitable for modification because of their method of manufacture. The heels may be of hollow plastic construction, and the soles may be attached to the uppers by adhesive or by injection moulding. A shoe, suitable for modification or use with an orthosis, is preferably of leather and welted construction, with laces. The heel should be broad, rather than narrow, and only of moderate height, that is not exceeding $1\frac{5}{8}$ inches (4.2 cm).

For convenience of discussion, pain in the foot is considered to arise from one or more of the following sites; ankle and sub-talar joints, heel, medial longitudinal arch, metatarsal arch and toes.

ANKLE AND SUB-TALAR JOINTS

Pain arising from the ankle or sub-talar joints may be relieved by limiting or preventing movement at the affected joints. This can be achieved by advising the patient to wear boots, by inserting an ankle stiffener or by adding a rocker bar to the sole of the shoe. A rocker bar is prescribed also following arthrodesis of the ankle to enable the patient to heel-toe smoothly.

Ankle stiffener
A boot restricts movement at the ankle joint. Further restriction can be obtained by adding an ankle stiffener. An ankle stiffener is made from metal or plastic. It extends upwards from the heel on the medial and/or lateral aspect of the ankle. It may be possible to remove the existing counter from a boot and replace it with a

new elongated one, but more commonly an ankle stiffener has to be added to the outside of the upper of the boot, its lower end being riveted to the existing counter.

Rocker bar

The apex of a rocker bar (Fig. 12.12) lies just behind and parallel to the line joining the first and fifth metatarsal heads. It differs from a metatarsal bar in that its anterior extension is longer, its overall length being up to $2\frac{1}{2}$ inches (5.6 cm).

As the sole of the shoe has been thickened by the addition of the rocker bar, it is sometimes necessary to raise the heel of the shoe by a similar amount. The heel of the other shoe may have to be raised also to balance the patient.

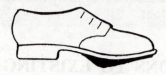

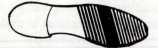

Fig. 12.12 Rocker bar for hallux rigidus. Note that the apex of the bar lies immediately behind and parallel to the line joining the first and fifth metatarsal heads, but that its anterior extension is longer than that of a metatarsal bar (Fig. 12.21).

Outside heel float

The lateral ligament of the ankle may be partially or completely ruptured following a severe inversion injury. This may result in the ankle being unstable and repeatedly suffering further inversion injuries.

In the absence of radiological evidence of increased talar tilt either with or without general anaesthesia, or if the patient should decline operative repair of the ligament, inversion injuries can be prevented by floating out the lateral side of the heel of the shoe (Fig. 12.13).

Fig. 12.13 Outside heel float. In addition an outside heel wedge can be added when weakness of the peroneal muscles is present.

Normally the first part of the heel of the shoe to strike the ground is situated about $\frac{1}{4}-\frac{1}{2}$ inch (0.6–1.25 cm) to the lateral side of the centre of the heel. By floating out the lateral side of the heel, the part of the heel which first strikes the ground is brought medially towards the mid-point of the now widened heel. This discourages the tendency to varus movement at the ankle and subtalar joints.

In muscle imbalance, when the peroneal muscles are weak, an outside heel float with possibly the addition of an outside heel wedge, an ankle stiffener or an ankle-foot orthosis — an inside below-knee iron with outside T-strap (see Ch. 11) — can be used to correct the varus deformity which occurs.

HEEL

Pain under the heel, for example from plantar fasciitis, may be relieved by fitting a horse-shoe shaped sponge rubber heel pad inside the shoe on a leather insole (Fig. 12.14). If the insole is not effective, it is possible to excavate the heel of a welted shoe and then to fill the cavity with sorbo rubber.

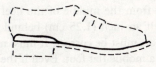

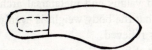

Fig. 12.14 Heel pad. Note the horse-shoe shape to the sponge rubber pad.

Pain over the *back of the heel* from an exostosis of the calcaneus can be relieved by removing the counter from the back of the shoe and inserting two small thick sponge rubber pads covered with chamois leather, one on each side of the exostosis (a tapered heel cushion).

MEDIAL LONGITUDINAL ARCH

Pain arising from the medial longitudinal arch of the foot may be due to foot strain (from prolonged unaccustomed standing, rapid increase in body weight, resumption of weight-bearing after a long period of bed rest), or degenerative changes in the tarsal and tarso-metatarsal joints. It is usually associated with flattening of the medial longitudinal arch and can be relieved by supporting that arch. This support can be obtained in a number of different ways.

Insoles

Valgus insoles
These are constructed commonly from felt or sponge rubber covered with leather and mounted on a firm leather insole (Fig. 12.15). Occasionally rigid arch supports made from metal or plastic are prescribed.

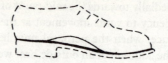

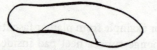

Fig. 12.15 Valgus insole, full length. The support extends from the middle of the heel forwards under the medial longitudinal arch to the metatarsal heads.

The support extends from the middle of the heel forward under the medial longitudinal arch to half an inch (1.25 cm) behind the metatarsal heads. The height of the arch support must be correct. It must not be too high for the rigid flat foot, or too low for a mobile flat foot. Even if the condition is unilateral it is advisable to prescribe a pair of insoles.

When marked flattening of the medial longitudinal arch is present attention must be paid to the metatarsal arch because support for both arches may be necessary. A combined valgus and metatarsal arch support may be prescribed also for pes cavus, so that the body weight is evenly distributed and pressure on the metatarsal heads is relieved.

Insoles may be either of full or three-quarter length. A full length insole is less likely to shift within the shoe with movement of the foot. It does, however, decrease the amount of space in which the toes can move, and therefore should not be prescribed if there is any tendency to hammer toe or claw toe deformity.

As an insole takes up space within a shoe it may be necessary to advise the patient to buy footwear half a size larger than he usually wears. Patients who have been prescribed insoles should be advised to wear them initially for only a short period during the day, gradually increasing the length of time until they are wearing them continuously.

Shoe alterations

Thomas heel

The front surface (heel breast) of a normal heel is slightly concave and runs transversely across the sole. In a Thomas heel (Fig. 12.16), the medial part of the heel breast is extended forward at least 1 inch (2.5 cm), at which point the front of the heel lies under the navicular bone. This gives support to the medial longitudinal arch.

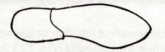

Fig. 12.16 Thomas heel.

Medial shank filler

Heavy patients sometimes depress the longitudinal arch of their shoes. This can be prevented and support for the medial longitudinal arch of the foot can be obtained by adding a medial shank filler, which fills in the gap between the ground and the under surface of the longitudinal arch of the shoe on the medial side. A medial shank filler extends from the medial part of the heel breast to the head of the first metatarsal where it is feathered to blend with the sole level with the break of the shoe (Fig. 12.17).

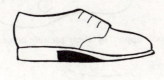

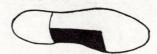

Fig. 12.17 Medial shank filler.

Medial heel and lateral sole wedges

This combination of wedges (cross wedging) produces a tendency to invert the heel and to evert the forefoot, which results in elevation of the medial longitudinal arch.

METATARSAL ARCH

Pain arising from the metatarsal arch region of the foot is usually due to the prominence of one or more of the central three metatarsal heads in the sole of the foot, associated with dorsal subluxation or dislocation of the respective metatarso-phalangeal joints. A hammer or claw toe deformity is usually present also. The latter may be associated with pes cavus. Other causes of metatarsalgia are Freiberg's disease of a metatarsal head, an interdigital neuroma, march fracture or disease such as rheumatoid arthritis. Symptoms can be alleviated by relieving pressure on the plantar aspect of the metatarsal heads.

Insoles, etc.

Metatarsal arch support

A metatarsal arch support consists of a pad of sponge rubber mounted on a firm leather insole and covered with leather. A single domed support (Fig. 12.18) will provide support for one or two of the middle metatarsal heads. When support for more than one or two metatarsal heads is indicated, a full width arch support is prescribed (Fig. 12.19).

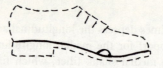

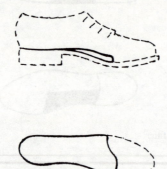

Fig. 12.18 Domed metatarsal support, to relieve pressure on one or two of the middle metatarsal heads.

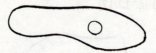

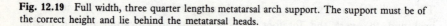

Fig. 12.19 Full width, three quarter lengths metatarsal arch support. The support must be of the correct height and lie behind the metatarsal heads.

A valgus and metatarsal arch support can be combined on one insole. As metatarsalgia is often associated with hammer or claw toe deformities, care must be taken before prescribing a metatarsal arch support on a full length insole. In such a situation a three-quarter length insole is preferable.

Metatarsal pad and garter
This consists of a pad of sponge rubber mounted on a broad elastic band, which is slipped over the foot (Fig. 12.20). It is useful in relieving mild metatarsalgia and has the additional advantage of allowing the patient to change his footwear without having to transfer any insoles.

Metatarsal arch supports must be of adequate thickness and must be

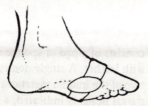

Fig. 12.20 Metatarsal pad and garter.

positioned correctly. This is very important. *They must lie behind* (not under) *the metatarsal heads*. Pressure on the metatarsal heads is reduced by the body weight being transferred through the necks of the metatarsals.

A new metatarsal arch support must be checked after it has been worn for one or two weeks. Prominent metatarsal heads tend to wear a depression in, or leave a clearer mark upon the insole. If the arch support is in the correct position neither of these two signs will be present. If these changes are present upon the insole, then the support is placed too far posteriorly, or is not high enough, and if present upon the arch support, then the support is placed too far forwards.

Shoe alterations

Metatarsal bar

Pressure on the metatarsal heads can be relieved also by placing a raised bar of leather or microcellular rubber across the sole of the shoe directly behind and parallel to the line between the first and fifth metatarsal heads (Fig. 12.21). The anterior and posterior extensions of the bar are feathered into the sole. The bar

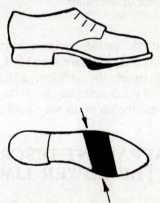

Fig. 12.21 Metatarsal bar for metatarsalgia. Note that the apex of the bar lies immediately behind and parallel to the line joining the first and fifth metatarsal heads.

takes the body weight behind the metatarsal heads and provides a rocker movement. The average height of the bar for adults is $\frac{5}{8}$ inch (1.5 cm). The disadvantage of this method is that the useful life of the bar is short due to wear, but it can be renewed easily without damage to the shoe.

TOES

Claw, hammer and mallet toes

Deformed toes may give rise to pain due to pressure upon them by the shoe. This pressure may be relieved by advising the patient to wear longer and wider shoes with a plain vamp; ensuring that the toe box is of adequate height; stretching the shoe over the deformed toes; inserting a balloon patch in the vamp where necessary; providing a metatarsal arch support if the deformities are mobile. It may be necessary, however, to prescribe surgical footwear to accommodate the deformities.

Hallux valgus and bunion

The pain from hallux valgus may be relieved by inserting a balloon patch in the vamp at the first metatarso-phalangeal joint, or by prescribing a pair of surgical shoes.

Hallux rigidus

The pain from hallux rigidus may be relieved by advising the patient to wear a thick, relatively stiff, soled pair of shoes, or by modifying the footwear so that dorsiflexion at the metatarso-phalangeal joint of the hallux is reduced or eliminated. This can be achieved in two ways.

1. The addition of a rocker bar to the sole of the shoe or boot (Fig. 12.12).

2. Stiffening the medial side of the sole of the shoe. In a shoe of welted construction, this can be achieved by elongating the shank so that it crosses the break of the shoe. An alternative method, in a shoe of non-welted construction, is to add an extra layer of leather (not microcellular rubber) to the sole of the shoe. The additional stiffness these procedures confer, prevents dorsiflexion at the metatarso-phalangeal joint of the hallux.

Toe block

Occasionally for multiple deformities, gangrene or infection, all the toes have to be amputated. Following this procedure a toe block is prescribed. It is made of sorbo rubber or Plastazote*. In addition, a light steel or high density polyethylene (Ortholene) shank extending from the heel to the toe of the shoe must be fitted, to prevent the tip of the shoe from curling upwards.

TRUE AND APPARENT DISCREPANCY IN LENGTH OF THE LOWER LIMBS

In clinical practice, the exact length of each lower limb is relatively unimportant. What is important is the difference in length which may exist between the two limbs. This difference in length may be true or apparent, or a combination of both.

TRUE DISCREPANCY IN LENGTH

True shortening of one lower limb is present when there is a decrease in the distance between the upper surface of the head of the femur and the lower surface of the calcaneus, compared with the other limb. This distance cannot be measured accurately by clinical means because of the deeply placed positions of the relevant bony points. Accurate measurement is possible only by taking a special radiograph — a scanograph — on which both lower limbs from the hips to the feet are shown alongside a scale.

For clinical purposes, the fixed bony points between which measurements are taken are the anterior superior iliac spine and the tip of the medial malleolus. It is accepted that the anterior superior iliac spine lies at a level proximal and lateral

---

*See Appendix.

to the upper surface of the head of the femur, and that a part of the talus and calcaneus lies distal to the tip of the medial malleolus. This means that destruction of the superior lip of the acetabulum, or upward dislocation of the head of the femur, will show as true shortening when in fact the distance between the upper surface of the head of the femur and the under surface of the calcaneus has not been altered. In addition loss of limb length from a compression fracture of the calcaneus will not be identified.

APPARENT DISCREPANCY IN LENGTH

Apparent discrepancy in length of the lower limbs is due to the presence of a fixed adduction or abduction deformity at one hip.

In normal standing, the lower limbs are parallel when seen from in front. To bring the lower limbs into a parallel position when a fixed adduction or abduction deformity is present at one hip, the pelvis is tilted and one knee is flexed. In the presence of a fixed adduction deformity, the anterior superior iliac spine on the same side is raised above the horizontal, causing apparent shortening of the ipsilateral limb. When a fixed abduction deformity is present, the anterior superior iliac spine on the opposite side is raised above the horizontal, causing apparent shortening of the contralateral limb (or apparent lengthening of the ipsilateral limb) (Fig. 12.22).

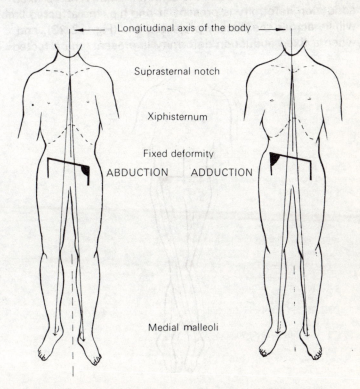

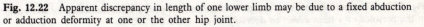

Fig. 12.22 Apparent discrepancy in length of one lower limb may be due to a fixed abduction or adduction deformity at one or the other hip joint.

The accurate measurement of apparent discrepancy in the length of the lower limb is unimportant clinically. What is important is that the detection of an apparent discrepancy in length indicates the presence of a fixed deformity at one hip.

HOW TO MEASURE THE LENGTHS OF THE LOWER LIMBS

True shortening

With the patient supine

— Stand on the right-hand side of the patient.

— Identify both anterior superior iliac spines and draw an imaginary line joining these two points.

— Project a second line distally from the centre and at right angles to the line joining the anterior superior iliac spines.

— Prior to measuring the true lengths, place the normal limb in a similar position to that of the affected limb. When a fixed adduction deformity is present at one hip, the affected limb will lie across the distally projected line (Fig. 12.23), and when a fixed abduction deformity is present, the affected

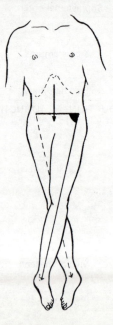

Fig. 12.23 The position in which the lower limbs must be placed when measuring for *true length* in the presence of a fixed *adduction deformity* at one (here the left) hip.

limb will lie some distance away from this line (Fig. 12.24).

— Grip one end of a tape measure between the tips of the *left* index finger and thumb, so that the thumb nail is at right angles to the upper surface of the tape measure.

— Slip the left thumb and tape measure in an upward direction until the pulp of the thumb, covered by the end of the tape measure, impinges upon the lower surface of the anterior superior iliac spine.

Identify the anterior superior iliac spine in this manner, as the presence of overlying mobile subcutaneous fatty tissue will make the accurate identification of the anterior superior iliac spine impossible by any other means.

— Maintain the left thumb in contact with the anterior superior iliac spine and lay the tape measure evenly along the medial border of the patella, and then slide the *right* thumb down the tape measure until it slips over the lower margin of the medial malleolus.

— Note the reading on the tape measure.

— Maintain the same grip on the tape measure with the left hand, and repeat the manoeuvre for the opposite limb.

— Any difference between the two measurements indicates the amount of true shortening present.

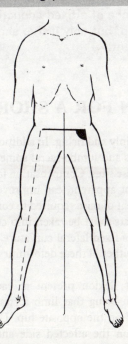

Fig. 12.24 The position in which the lower limbs must be placed when measuring for *true length* in the presence of a fixed *abduction deformity* at one (here the left) hip.

With the patient standing

— Stand the patient erect with both kness fully extended.
— Identify both anterior superior iliac spines. The anterior superior iliac spine on the side of the shorter limb will lie at a lower level.
— Place wooden blocks of varying thickness under the foot of the shorter limb until the anterior superior iliac spines lie on a horizontal plane.
— The total height of the wooden blocks used equals the difference in limb length.

Apparent shortening

The apparent lengths of the lower limbs are measured from a fixed median point, such as the xiphisternum or suprasternal notch, to the tips of the medial malleoli.
— Lie the patient supine.
— Ignoring the position of the pelvis, arrange the lower limbs evenly about the longitudinal axis of the trunk, with only 3–4 inches (7.5–10 cm) between the medial malleoli (Fig. 12.22).
— Measure the distance from the xiphisternum or suprasternal notch to the lower margin of each malleolus, handling the tape measure as described above.
— A difference between the measurements for each lower limb indicates the presence of a fixed adduction or abduction deformity at one hip, but only if true shortening or lengthening is absent.

COMPENSATION FOR A SHORT LOWER LIMB

A short leg gait can be ungainly and tiring. In addition it can increase the stresses imposed upon the hip joints and lumbo-sacral spine and therefore contribute to the occurrence of pain at these sites. Compensation for inequality in length of the lower limbs, whether true or apparent, can improve function.

Before determing the height of raise required to compensate for shortening of a lower limb, a number of facts must be taken into consideration.

1. Does the patient have a fixed lateral curvature of the spine, or fixed pelvic obliquity? The presence of either of these deformities will influence the degree of pelvic tilt which can occur.

2. What is the range of flexion present at each hip? When one hip is arthrodesed, the patient can bring that limb forward during walking only by swinging the pelvis forward on the opposite hip. Unless sufficient clearance is allowed between the foot on the affected side and the ground, this will be impossible. Any raise supplied must be such that the affected limb is effectively $\frac{1}{2}$ inch (1.25 cm) shorter than the other limb to give sufficient clearance.

3. What is the range of flexion present at each knee? Again any raise supplied must allow sufficient clearance — $\frac{1}{2}$ inch (1.25 cm) — to bring the affected limb forward.

4. What degree of fixed equinus (plantar flexion) of the ankle or forefoot is present? The degree of these deformities will determine the heights of the raises under the heel, the tread (metatarsal heads) and the toes.

5. What degree of mobility exists at the ankle and in the forefoot? As much equinus of the ankle and forefoot (pitch) as possible is allowed. This improves the appearance and decreases the weight of the footwear.

6. Is dorsiflexion at the metatarso-phalangeal joint of the hallux limited? Limitation of movement at this joint influences the amount of equinus of the ankle and forefoot which can be allowed. If too great a degree of equinus is allowed, the metatarso-phalangeal joint of the hallux will be forced into dorsiflexion. This may give rise to pain.

CALCULATION OF THE AMOUNT OF RAISE REQUIRED

It is rarely necessary to compensate for the first half an inch (1.25 cm) of shortening, as this amount can be accommodated easily by tilting the pelvis.

Although the theoretical height of the heel raise required to compensate for any shortening can be calculated by subtracting half an inch (1.25 cm) from the difference in length of the lower limbs measured with the patient supine, this method is unlikely to be satisfactory. All patients who require compensation for shortening must be measured in the standing position. In this position the height of the heel raise, and the degree of allowable equinus of the ankle and forefoot necessary to compensate for any true or apparent shortening, *which is comfortable to the patient,* can be determined. The comfort of the patient is much more important than any theoretical calculation.

— Stand the patient erect with both knees fully extended.
— Insert wooden blocks under the foot of the shorter limb. Blocks equal to the theoretical height of the required raise can be used initially.
— Tell the patient to mark time.
— Vary the thickness of the wooden blocks under the heel and tread until the patient is comfortable. Remind the patient to mark time between each variation in thickness of the wooden blocks.
— The ultimate thickness of the wooden blocks under the heel and tread equals the height of the raise required at these sites.

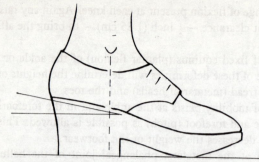

Fig. 12.25 The height of a heel raise is measured in front of the centre of the heel, in line with the medial malleolus. Note that the heel raise must be higher posteriorly than anteriorly.

Note: The height of the heel raise is measured anterior to the *centre* of the heel of the shoe, that is, in line with the medial malleolus (Fig. 12.25). This means that when a raise is added to the heel of a shoe, the thickness of the posterior border of the heel must be greater than that of the anterior border, otherwise the under surface of the sole and heel will not make simultaneous contact with the ground when standing, and all the stress will be taken by the anterior border of the heel.

As it is necessary to provide a rocker action for walking, the height of the raise must decrease towards the toe (Fig. 12.26). The height of the raise at the toe will depend upon that at the tread. If this is large, the tapering must be more.

Occasionally after giving a patient a raise determined in the above way, the gait pattern may still be poor. Do not over-compensate for shortening to try to improve a gait pattern in the presence of adequate compensation for shortening, as the poor gait pattern may be due to weakness of the spinal or abdominal muscles.

TYPES OF RAISES EMPLOYED

Outside raise

If the foot is normal, the raise can be added to ordinary footwear. Sensible footwear is essential. Certain types of footwear are unsuitable for the addition of a raise, for example:

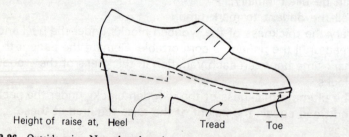

Height of raise at, Heel   Tread   Toe

Fig. 12.26 Outside raise. Note that the raise tapers towards the toe to aid walking.

Shoes with heels exceeding 2 inches (5.0 cm) in height.

Court shoes. The addition of a raise to a court shoe causes loss of flexibility of the shoes with the result that the patient's heel tends to come out of the shoe.

Shoes with welded rubber soles and heels, as it is difficult to remove the original sole.

Soft suede shoes or boots are not suitable for a raise in excess of $1\frac{1}{2}$ inches (3.75 cm).

When the required raise is $\frac{1}{4}-\frac{3}{4}$ inch (0.6–2.0 cm), the heel and if necessary the sole can be raised by adding to the surface of the existing heel and sole. Microcellular rubber is used for the raise in preference to leather, as it is lighter, more flexible and wears better.

When a heel raise of more than three-quarters of an inch (2.0 cm) is required, the existing sole and heel are removed and layers of cork are added to obtain the required height. The cork layers are shaped and covered with leather similar to that of the shoe. The original sole and heel are reattached if possible, or if not, a new sole and heel are made (Figs 12.26, 12.27).

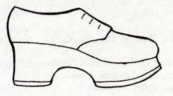

Fig. 12.27 Outside raise — arched.

Inside raise

When a foot is deformed or of an odd size, surgical footwear must be made. In these cases, all or part of the raise may be concealed within the upper. This is known as an inside raise (Fig. 12.28). The maximum height for an inside raise is usually $3\frac{1}{2}$ inches (8.0 cm) at the heel, with 2 inches (5.0 cm) at the tread, and approximately 1 inch (2.5 cm) at the toe. If a larger raise than this is required, the additional height is obtained by adding an outside raise.

When the required raise is more than $3\frac{1}{2}$ inches (8.0 cm), the cork raise can be arched and bridge waisted. The bridge, which must be strong and perhaps reinforced with a steel plate, prevents the heel and tread raises from splaying out on walking (Fig. 12.29).

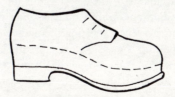

Fig. 12.28 Inside raise in a surgical shoe.

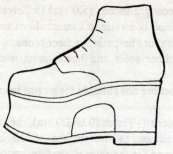

Fig. 12.29 Outside raise, arched and bridge waisted.

As has already been mentioned, as much equinus of the ankle and forefoot as possible is allowed. However, in such a situation the heel platform must be flat to prevent the patient's foot from sliding down the slope and the patient's toes impinging against the tip of the shoe.

REFERENCES

Shaw, P. (1976) The Surgical Boot. In Murdoch, G. (ed.) *The Advances in Orthotics*, p. 93. London: Arnold.
Staros, A. (1976) A Programme for Provision of Orthopaedic Shoes. In Murdoch, G. (ed). *The Advances in Orthotics*, p. 101. London: Arnold.
Tuck, W.H. (1971) Personal communcation.

13.

Splinting and casting materials

In the last few years, there has been a rapid proliferation of casting materials available to the orthopaedic surgeon, and more will be developed with the aid of modern technology. The following comments are intended to assist in the understanding and use of these different materials.

HISTORY OF CASTING MATERIALS

The urge to immobilise a fractured limb is basic. Hippocrates, in about 350 BC, used bandages stiffened by waxes and resins to treat fractures, and Rhazes, born in 860 AD, in Arabia, used lime and egg white. In 1756, Cheselden, an English surgeon, used bandages soaked in egg white and flour to form a cast which could be split longitudinally to allow it to be tightened or loosened.

In the 18th century, in the Turkish empire, plaster-of-Paris was used in the treatment of fractures. The limb was enclosed in a case of plaster and any space which appeared as swelling subsided, was filled by pouring plaster cream through a hole in the cast. Hubenthal, in 1816, improved upon this by mixing plaster-of-Paris and minced blotting paper in equal proportions. In 1828 in Berlin, Koyl and Kluge used a wooden box in which they rested the injured limb. They then poured plaster-of-Paris cream into the box until the limb was nearly covered. This resulted in a rather cumbersome cast.

Plaster-of-Paris bandages were first used by Matthysen, a Dutch military surgeon, in 1852. They were made by rubbing dry plaster-of-Paris powder into coarsely woven cotton bandages, which were then soaked in water before being applied. They had to be freshly prepared before use (Monro, 1935).

This was the principle of all plaster-of-Paris bandages used until they became available commercially in 1931. Various substances are added now to improve the handling characteristics of the bandages, allowing more thorough and even wetting, reducing the loss of plaster during soaking and accelerating the setting time.

Although some plastics were developed as casting materials in the 1950s, it is only within the last few years that this development has been really successful with the production of a large range of materials with widely differing properties suitable for specific purposes.

ORTHOPAEDIC USE OF CASTS

In traumatic and orthopaedic surgery, the casting material is wrapped around the patient's limb or trunk and held there while it hardens. The cast which results accurately follows all the contours of the encased part of the body, and will support that part firmly and evenly if left in place, or provide an exact negative mould if removed.

The use of casts in traumatic and orthopaedic surgery can be summarised as follows:

To support fractured bones, controlling movement of the fragments and resting the damaged soft tissues.

To stabilise and rest joints where there has been ligamentous injury.

To support and immobilise joints and limbs post-operatively until healing has occurred after for example, the repair of nerves or tendons.

To correct a deformity by wedging the cast or the application of serial or turnbuckle casts.

To ensure rest of infected tissues.

To make a removable splint to aid mobilisation or prevent deformity.

To render it difficult for a patient to remove dressings or tamper with a wound.

To make a negative mould of a part of the body, as a preliminary step in the accurate construction of orthotic or prosthetic appliances.

To make a cast of part of a patient's body upon which an orthotic or prosthetic appliance can be constructed, a negative mould of that part of the body must first be made. To do this a plaster-of-Paris cast is applied over a single layer of stockinette after the skin has been greased to help in the removal of the cast. A strip of lead or plastic may be placed on the skin where the cast is to be cut to enable it to be removed. When the cast is dry, it is marked and then carefully removed, before being reassembled using the marks to ensure accuracy. A positive cast is then made by pouring plaster-of-Paris cream into the negative mould which has been coated inside with a releasing agent. Once the positive cast has set, the negative mould is removed, leaving an exact replica of part of the patient. In the construction of the orthotic or prosthetic appliance, tools, processes and materials can be used which could not be used on the patient's actual limb, and in addition the work can be carried out in a workshop remote from the hospital. Occasionally modern plastic materials are used for the original cast which can be used as part of the finished appliance, without the need for any intermediate stages.

MATERIALS AVAILABLE FOR CASTING

The materials which are used for making casts on a patient are either:
1. Plaster-of-Paris.
2. Plaster-of-Paris with melamine resins.
3. Materials which undergo polymerisation
   a. Water activated
   b. Non-water activated.
4. Low-temperature thermoplastics.

The orthotist can use high-temperature thermoplastics and thermo-setting plastics to make orthoses moulded on a positive plaster cast, but these materials cannot be used directly on the patient.

PLASTER-OF-PARIS

Plaster-of-Paris has been used since early Egyptian times for decorating walls, but it is only since the 1800s that it has been used for orthopaedic casts. It is made from gypsum, a naturally occurring mineral. The name, plaster-of-Paris, is said to stem from an accident to a house built on a deposit of gypsum, near Paris. The house burnt down. When rain fell on the baked mud of the floors, it was noted that footprints in the mud set rock-hard. This led to the rediscovery of the practice of heating gypsum to make a smooth covering for walls. When Henry III visited Paris in 1254, he admired the smooth whiteness of the walls and popularised the use of plaster-of-Paris for walls in England. The Romans had used plaster to cover their walls during the occupation of Britain, but the technique had been lost (Smith & Nephew, 1967).

To make plaster-of-Paris, gypsum is heated to drive off water. When water is added to the resulting powder, the original mineral reforms and heat is released.

$$2(CaSO_4 . 2H_2O) + Heat \rightleftharpoons 2(CaSO_4 . \tfrac{1}{2} H_2O) + 3H_2O$$

Calcium sulphate dihydrate + Heat $\rightleftharpoons$ Calcium sulphate hemi-hydrate + Water

Modern plaster-of-Paris bandages are made by grinding gypsum and then heating it in a steam pressure autoclave. The powder is suspended in a volatile solvent with the various additives to improve the handling characteristics. The resultant slurry is coated onto the special interlock woven cloth, called leno. The solvent is removed in a drying oven after which the bandages are cut, rolled and packed in moisture-resistant containers.

Closely conforming casts can be made by using plaster-of-Paris bandages prepared on an elastic cloth instead of the usual cotton cloth. The bandages can stretch when wet to follow the shape of the limb, but once set they are the same as ordinary plaster casts. Orthoflex* is such a type of bandage.

PLASTER-OF-PARIS WITH MELAMINE RESINS

Melamine synthetic resin was mixed with plaster-of-Paris to form water-resistant casts in the 1950s (Morrison, 1953; Maudsley, 1955). The resin sets after contact with water and reinforces the plaster-of-Paris bandage. With modifications, this form of casting material has continued in use to the present day (Zoroc*; Cellamin*).

MATERIALS WHICH UNDERGO POLYMERISATION

These form a complex group of materials which are undergoing continuous development. Several of them are prepared in a form which requires the addition of water to convert them to their rigid state, whereas others are polymerised by different agents.

---

*See Appendix.

Table 13.1

Name	Presentation	Preparation	Equipment	Set	Load-Bearing	Strength/Weight	Stiffness	Flammability	Remouldable	X-Ray Clarity	Mess	Shelf-Life	Comments
Plaster-of-Paris													
Gypsona*	Cotton bandages spread with plaster-of-Paris	Water at 25–30°C	Bucket	4–5 min	48 h	Moderate	Rigid	Nil	No	Relatively opaque	Considerable	2–3 years in a dry store	Dust if saw used for removal
Cellona*	Cotton bandages spread with plaster-of-Paris	Water at 20–25°C	Bucket	3½ min	48 h	Moderate	Rigid	Nil	No	Relatively opaque	Considerable	2 years in a dry store. Manufacture date on box	Dust if saw used for removal
Orthoflex*	Elastic bandage spread with plaster-of-Paris	Water at 29°C	Bucket	5 min	48 h	Moderate	Rigid	Nil	No	Relatively opaque	Considerable	3 years foil wrapped	Dust if saw used for removal
Mixtures of plaster-of-Paris and melamine resin													
Zoroc*	Cotton bandage spread with plaster-of-Paris & melamine resin	Water at 29°C	Bucket & gloves	5–8 min	1 h	Fairly light & strong	Rigid	Nil	No	More translucent than plaster	Very little	3 years foil wrapped	Small amount of formaldehyde
Cellamin*	Cotton bandage spread with plaster-of-Paris & melamine resin	Water at 20°C	Bucket & gloves or hand-cream	3½–4½ min	24 h	Fairly light & strong	Rigid	Nil	No	More translucent than plaster	Very little	2 years foil wrapped	Small amount of formaldehyde

Table 13.1 (continued)

Water-activated polymerisable materials

Name	Presentation	Preparation	Equipment	Set	Load-Bearing	Strength/Weight	Stiffness	Flammability	Remould-able	X-Ray Clarity	Mess	Shelf-Life	Comments
Bayacast* (Cuttercast in USA)	Cotton bandage with polyurethane prepolymer	Water at about 21°C	Bucket & gloves	3–5 min	30 min	Very light & strong	Slightly flexible	Flammable, as clothing	No	Translucent at 'skin' exposure	None	15 months foil wrapped. Expiry date shown	Heat when applied if cast thick
Scotchcast*	Knitted fibreglass bandage with polyurethane pre-polymer	Water at 18–24°C	Bucket & gloves with hand-cream	5–10 min	30 min	Light & very strong	Almost rigid	Flammable, as clothing	No	Transluscent	None	12 months foil wrapped	Hard to cut
Scotchflex*	Conforming knitted fibreglass bandage with polyurethane prepolymer	Water at 18–24°C	Bucket & gloves with hand-cream	5–10 min	30 min	Light & strong	Slightly flexible	Flammable, as clothing	No	Translucent	None	12 months foil wrapped	Easier to cut than Scotchcast
Crystona*	Polyester/cotton bandage with acrylic polymer & glass	Water at 20°C	Bucket & gloves	11 min	60 min	Light & strong	Almost rigid	Nil	No	More transluscent than plaster	A little powder	Over 2 years	Hard to cut with saw
Deltalite*§ fabric	Cotton/polyester knitted bandage with polyurethane prepolymer	Water at 21–27°C	Bucket & gloves	7 min	20 min	Light & strong	Fairly rigid	Flammable, as clothing	No	Transluscent	None	2 years foil wrapped	
Deltalite*§ glass	Knitted fibreglass bandage with polyurethane prepolymer	Water at 21–27°C	Bucket & gloves	7 min	20 min	Light & very strong	Almost rigid	Flammable, as clothing	No	Translucent	None	2 years foil wrapped	

Table 13.1 (continued)

Non-water-activated polymerisable materials

Name	Presentation	Preparation	Equipment	Set	Load-Bearing	Strength/Weight	Stiffness	Flammability	Remouldable	X-Ray Clarity	Mess	Shelf-Life	Comments
Lighticast II*	Fibreglass bandage with photosensitive vinyl-toluene resin	Bandages moulded & set under ultraviolet light	U-V light source of approved type & gloves	3 min	3 min	Light & very strong	Slightly flexible	Less flammable than clothing	No	Translucent	None	Over 3 years	Odour
Glassona*	Knitted bandage of glass and cellulose acetate fibres	Acetone solvent	Safe container for solvent & gloves	15 min	24 hours	Light & strong	Slightly flexible	Highly flammable	No	Translucent	Moderate	Over 3 years	Skin irritant
Neofract*	Two-part polyurethane with pre-fabricated zipped 'garments'	Machine mixed and poured into 'garments'. Self moulding	Mixing machine, roller and range of 'garments'	5–10 min	30 min	Light & strong	Fairly rigid	Less flammable than clothing	Limited remoulding at 100°C	Much more translucent than plaster	Some	Over 1 year	
Fibreglass*†	Commercial DIY glassfibre kits	Resin mixed with catalyst and spread on glass cloth	Mixing jar, gloves, protective sheets	10 min	30–60 min	Light & strong	Fairly rigid	Flammable	No	More translucent than plaster	Considerable	1–2 years	Odour, adheres to skin. Hard to cut. Impermeable

Table 13.1 (continued)

Name	Presentation	Preparation	Equipment	Set	Load-Bearing	Strength/Weight	Stiffness	Flammability	Remouldable	X-Ray Clarity	Mess	Shelf-Life	Comments
Thermoplastics													
Hexcelite*	Open mesh thermoplastic bandage and sheet	Heat in water at 71°C	Thermostatic water bath. Hot air gun	3–4 min	15 min	Light & strong	Slightly flexible	Flammable, as clothing	Yes	Translucent with 50% exposure for plaster	None	Indefinite	No hazards
Orthoplast*	Isoprene rubber sheets. Plain or perforated	Heat in water at 72–77°C	Hot water bath	5–8 min	30 min	Light & strong	Slightly flexible	Flammable, as clothing	Yes	Translucent	None	Indefinite	No hazards
Plastazote*	Closed cell cross-linked polyethylene foam sheets												
Low density polymer	PO73 (pink) low density foam sheets. 40–50 kg/m³	Heat in an oven at 140°C for 20 s for each mm thickness	Oven with enclosed heating elements	75% of heating time	20 s for each mm thickness	Light & fairly strong	Flexible	Flammable, melts with burning drips	Yes	Translucent	None	Indefinite	
	PO77 (white) heavier density foam sheets, 65–75 kg/m³	ditto	ditto	ditto	ditto	ditto	ditto	ditto	ditto	ditto	ditto	ditto	
High density polymer	HO62 (black) high density foam sheets. 90–110 kg/m³	Heat in an oven at 140°C for 1 min for each mm thickness	ditto & gloves	ditto	1 min for each mm thickness	Light & strong	Fairly rigid	ditto	ditto	ditto	ditto	ditto	When moulding on the patient use a layer of low density foam before applying high density foam

* See Appendix
† Note that the authors do not recommend fibreglass for use in orthopaedic casts but recognise that it may have applications in certain circumstances
§ Available only in USA

Water activated

These are chemicals which are coated onto fabric or glass cloth to form bandages. Contact with water initiates polymerisation so that the bandages set (Baycast★; Scotchcast★; Crystona★).

Non-water activated

The materials in this group may be coated onto fabric and be activated by a chemical solvent or by the addition of a catalyst. Ultraviolet light, of a wavelength not harmful to the eyes, is the activating agent for one photosensitive resin (Lightcast II★). Another material consists of a two-part polyurethane that foams when mixed, and becomes a self-moulding cast when poured into a double-walled, fabric tube pre-shaped to fit different parts of the body (Neofract★).

LOW-TEMPERATURE THERMOPLASTICS

These are inert plastics which become pliable when heated and harden when cooled. Theoretically the cycle can be repeated indefinitely, but in practice it is restricted to modifying casts or splints rather than re-using the material for different patients. The temperature to which these materials have to be heated exceeds that which can be tolerated by the skin, but since they are poor conductors of heat they do not cause burns as long as the surface is dry and has been allowed to cool slightly after the material has been removed from the oven or water bath. These materials are prepared as sheets (Orthoplast★; Plastazote★) or open mesh bandages (Hexcelite★). In practice there does not seem to be a problem from softening of the casts when the patient stands close to a heat source, as sufficient heat passes through the walls of the cast to cause the patient to move away before the cast becomes soft.

CHOICE OF MATERIAL FOR SPECIFIC PURPOSES

The material chosen for any particular cast will depend upon a number of different factors — the reason for the cast, the experience of the user, the strength which is required in the cast, the duration for which the cast will be required, the likely exposure to water or soiling, the need for lightness, the likely need to modify the cast, the expense of the casting material.

It is likely that plaster-of-Paris will remain the standard material for most casts and especially those used in the initial management of new fractures. It is familiar to all doctors as well as being cheap and the least demanding of materials to apply. It is permeable to air and allows blood, pus and odour to pass through to the surface and become obvious. Very accurate casting can be obtained with it,

---

*See Appendix.

and its comfort and appearance can be excellent when it is skilfully applied.

When a patient is frail, a light-weight cast may be best, and may enable the patient to be mobilised rather than remain confined to bed. A light-weight cast may also be used in the later stages of management of a fracture in younger patients. A plastic material is chosen. Those available in a bandage form are easier to mould, but this is still more difficult than with plaster-of-Paris.

Many plaster-of-Paris casts are damaged by patients walking on them before they have thoroughly dried. These have to be replaced with the resultant waste of time and materials. Plastic materials which achieve their maximum final strength quickly are ideal for weight-bearing casts. Their ability to withstand early weight-bearing reduces the chance of damage, and may allow a patient to be allowed home rather than stay in hospital just because he is unable to walk non-weight bearing with crutches.

Casts frequently are needed for several weeks or months in the management of orthopaedic conditions in children. Plaster-of-Paris casts are easily damaged by children, but this damage can be avoided if a layer of tough, water-resistant synthetic material is applied over the plaster-of-Paris. Many of these synthetic materials can be used also to repair damaged casts, the resulting repair being lighter and stronger than if plaster-of-Paris had been used. However, casts must be repaired, rather than be replaced, only if it is certain that the inner layers of the cast have not been disturbed. If the inner layers of the cast have become roughened or irregular, repair of the cast can lead to discomfort and even the development of a pressure sore.

Expensive plastic casting materials generally are not used for casts which may have to be removed for remanipulation or to allow frequent examination.

A non-inflammable cast should be considered if a patient is likely to be exposed to naked flames. All forms of padding used under casts are inflammable, as is most clothing. The authors however, have been unable to find any authenticated account of injuries being caused by a cast catching fire.

Some new casting materials can be remoulded by applying heat or more solvent. This can be an advantage where it is necessary to relieve pressure over bony prominences, or the shape requires to be changed as swelling subsides.

Radiographs of high resolution cannot be taken through plaster-of-Paris. Some synthetic casts however are almost transparent to X-rays.

Potential allergy or other health hazards to both the patient and the user must be considered when choosing and using casting materials. Gloves frequently have to be worn when using some of the newer casting materials, both to ease handling of the materials as well as to protect the user from allergic skin reactions.

A few materials incorporating glass (Crystona*; Fibreglass*; Scotchcast*) are hard to cut and may require specially hardened cutting tools or blades if these are not to be quickly blunted.

At present the ideal casting material does not exist. If it did it might have the following properties — be suitable for direct application to the patient, be easy to mould, be non-toxic to both the patient and user, be unaffected by fluids such as

---

*See Appendix.

water, be transparent to X-rays, be easy to modify, be quick setting, be easy to remove, be able to transmit air, odour, water, pus, be strong but light in weight, be non-inflammable, be non-messy in application and removal, have a long shelf-life and be cheap.

REFERENCES

Maudsley, R.H. (1955) Resin-impregnated plasters. *Lancet,* **i,** 847.

Monro, J.K. (1935) The history of plaster-of-Paris in the treatment of fractures. *British Journal of Surgery,* **23,** 257.

Morrison, J.B. (1953) Melamine resin in the making of plaster casts. *Lancet,* **ii,** 1317.

Smith & Nephew Ltd (1967) *The History and Function of Plaster-of-Paris in Surgery.* Welwyn Garden City, Herts.

14.

Plaster-of-Paris casts

Plaster-of-Paris casts can be responsible for the development of serious complications.

IMPAIRMENT OF CIRCULATION

A limb which has been fractured, or upon which an operation has been performed, will always swell to a greater or lesser degree because of haemorrhage from the bone and surrounding traumatised soft tissue, and because of reactionary tissue oedema. If such a limb has been encased in a plaster cast the swelling can result in an appreciable increase in pressure within the cast, and cause a reduction in or the obliteration of the blood supply of the muscles and nerves. An increase in the pressure within a fascial compartment of the limb in the absence of a plaster cast can have the same result. *This impairment of the circulation can occur in the presence of distal peripheral pulses.* Ischaemia causes tissue death and subsequent fibrosis. Joint contracture, muscle paralysis and altered cutaneous sensibility may develop and cause considerable permanent impairment of the future function of that limb.

Patients who have sustained a fracture or undergone an operation commonly suffer pain. This pain rapidly and progressively decreases over the following two to three days. The persistence, the increase, or the recurrence of pain in an injured limb may herald the onset of circulatory impairment, or the development of a pressure sore.

Circulatory embarrassment or the development of a pressure sore is accompanied by severe pain. It is important to remember that patients do not always complain of pain to the attending doctor for varying reasons. *Every patient who has a plaster cast applied must be directly questioned as to the presence of pain. Do not wait for the patient to complain of pain — it may then be too late.*

TO PREVENT VASCULAR COMPLICATIONS

— Do not apply an unpadded plaster cast to a recently fractured limb. Many fractures can be adequately immobilised initially by the application over padding of a partly encircling plaster slab, the slab being retained by an encircling bandage. If a complete plaster cast must be used to maintain position, the plaster must be applied over padding. Preferably the plaster cast then should be split throughout its length.

— After an operation, always apply a well padded plaster cast, or split a lightly padded cast throughout its length.

— Elevate the encased limb so that gravity can assist the venous return from the limb.

— Encourage active finger and toe movements, again to assist the venous return.

— **Keep a frequent and careful check upon the state of the circulation in the affected limb.**

1. Enquire about the presence and site of any pain. *Never ignore the complaint of pain,* as even a fussy patient can develop circulatory embarrassment or a pressure sore.

2. Examine the fingers or toes for swelling. Swelling may be due to venous obstruction, dependency of the injured limb, insufficient active exercise or a combination of all three.

3. Compare the state of the capillary circulation, especially in the nail beds, in the injured limb with that in the uninjured limb. Blanching on pressure should be followed by a quick return of colour on release of the pressure. The colour should be pink. Blueness of the extremities suggests venous obstruction. It should disappear on elevation of the limb. White and cold fingers or toes suggest arterial obstruction.

4. The peripheral pulses may be obscured by the cast, but where possible palpate them and compare with the uninjured limb. Remember that circulatory embarrassment can be present even when the distal pulses are palpable.

5. Examine the extremities for the presence of altered skin sensibility — hypoaesthesia.

6. Test the ease and range of active and passive movement of the fingers and toes. Pain on passive extension of the fingers or toes is strongly indicative of ischaemia of the flexor muscle groups.

If there is evidence of impairment of the circulation in a limb, the plaster cast must be split at once throughout its lengh, or removed completely. If impairment is due to a rise of pressure within a fascial compartment, then the limb must be decompressed immediately. Remember that the splitting or removal of a plaster cast may not be sufficient; the limb may also need to be decompressed. The delay of a few hours may have disastrous consequences. A good rule is if in doubt split the plaster cast: it is better to split a cast unnecessarily and possibly lose the position, than to run the risk of ischaemic changes occurring in a limb.

In general a lower limb cast is split along the front, and an upper limb cast along the ulnar of flexor surface. How to split a plaster cast is described later.

PRESSURE SORES

Pressure sores can develop under a plaster cast due to irregularity of the inner surface of the cast, insufficient padding especially over bony prominences, the presence of foreign bodies such as coins or matchsticks between the cast and the skin, or from the chafing of the skin by the rough edges of a crack in the cast. The development of pressure sores can be prevented by the careful application of adequate padding, by the avoidance of varying tension in a roll of padding or plaster as it is being applied, and by the avoidance of localised areas of pressure by fingers or thumb while the plaster is wet. With regard to the latter, a wet cast must be held only in the palm of the hand, so that pressure is spread over a wide area. In addition a wet cast must be supported throughout its length on a pillow until it is dry, to avoid direct pressure on an underlying bony prominence, such as the heel or the point of the elbow.

DIAGNOSIS OF THE PRESENCE OF A PRESSURE SORE

1. Pain
Pressure sores are painful initially. The pain will decrease when full thickness skin ulceration occurs. If a patient complains of pain under a plaster cast, which is not referable to the fracture or operation, the presence of a pressure sore must be suspected.

2. Fretfulness
Especially in children. Children may be too young to complain of localised pain.

3. Disturbed sleep
This again particularly applies to children.

4. Rise in temperature

5. Recurrence of swelling of the fingers and toes
Once the initial swelling has subsided.

6. The presence of an offensive smell

7. Discharge
A discharge may present either from under the edge of the cast or by the appearance of a stain on a previously clean area of the cast.

By the time the patient exhibits a rise in temperature, or there is a recurrence of swelling of the fingers or toes, or an offensive smell or discharge is noted, full thickness skin ulceration with possibly necrosis of the underlying fat and muscle will have occurred. The presence of a pressure sore must be diagnosed before this state is reached.

If the presence of a pressure sore is suspected, the skin in that area must be examined immediately either by cutting a window, or by removing the cast altogether (these procedures are described in detail later). It is better to lose position rather than allow a pressure sore to develop.

INSTRUCTIONS TO AN OUT-PATIENT WEARING A PLASTER CAST

Only a small number of patients who have had a plaster cast applied are admitted to hospital. The vast majority are treated as out-patients.

Before any patient is allowed to leave hospital, the circulation in the encased limb must be checked and found to be satisfactory. In addition the patient must be given the following instructions both verbally and in writing.

1. Time and place of his next out-patient attendance which should be within the next 24 hours.
2. How to recognise, and what to do about possible complications.
3. What precautions to take with regard to the plaster cast.

The following is a suggested sheet of instructions to give to a patient:

Instructions to patients in a plaster cast

IMPORTANT

Report back to the hospital immediately at any time of the day or night if
You get increased pain, or pins and needles in the plastered limb.
Your fingers or toes become blue, white, badly swollen or numb.
You are unable to move your fingers or toes.
You loose any object, such as a coin or pencil, under the plaster cast.

Do not rest the plaster cast on a firm surface.
Do not hang the splinted limb down unless the limb is in active use.
Use the splinted limb as much as possible. Move your fingers and toes, and all other joints not immobilised by the plaster cast, a number of times every hour.
Keep the plaster cast dry.
Report back to the hospital if the plaster cast becomes loose, cracked or soft.

The application of the different plaster casts used in the treatment of fractures and other conditions is not described. This is well described in other books (*Plaster-of-Paris Technique; Gypsona Technique; Orthopaedic Nursing*).

The following procedures are described:
Removing a plaster cast.
Pre-operative preparation of a limb immobilised in a plaster cast.
Cutting a window in a plaster cast.
Splitting a plaster cast.
Wedging a plaster cast.

REMOVING A PLASTER CAST

A plaster cast used for the external immobilisation of a fracture will be removed after a certain number of weeks, to determine the state of union clinically and radiologically. When a plaster cast is removed, it is important that the skin of the limb is not damaged, the patient is not subjected to pain, and control of the fracture is maintained until it is decided that the cast can be discarded.

The plaster cast can be cut with plaster shears or with an electric plaster saw (e.g. Zimmer). Generally shears are used for children, small casts, and casts on the upper limbs. *The electric plaster saw must not be used on unpadded casts.* It may be used with great care when there is only stockinette under the cast.

HOW TO USE AN ELECTRIC PLASTER SAW (Fig. 14.1)

The cutting blade of an electric plaster saw does not rotate. It oscillates, and will damage the skin only if it is drawn along the limb or if the skin is adherent to the underlying bone and therefore not mobile.

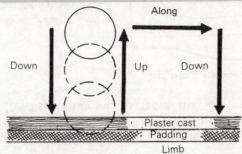

Fig. 14.1 The correct way to use an electric plaster saw.

- Switch on the saw.
- Demonstrate to the patient that the saw will not cut skin, by placing the oscillating blade in contact with your own hand.
- With light pressure apply the cutting blade to the plaster cast, keeping a finger under the neck of the saw to control the depth of the cut. In this way it is easy to feel when the saw has cut through the cast.
- Remove the blade from the cut formed in the cast.
- Reapply the cutting blade at a slightly higher or lower level.
- Repeat these separate and distinct movements until the cast has been divided along its length.
  Do not draw the cutting blade of an electric plaster saw along the limb, otherwise the skin will be cut. Take particular care when there is a blood-soaked dressing under the cast.
  Do not hold the electric saw with wet hands, or allow the saw or the lead to the saw to get wet.

HOW TO REMOVE A PLASTER CAST (Fig. 14.2)

- Determine if the cast is padded.
- Choose a line along which to cut the cast, avoiding any bony prominences, to reduce the risk of skin damage. For a lower limb cast, the line must pass in front of the lateral malleolus and behind the medial malleolus.

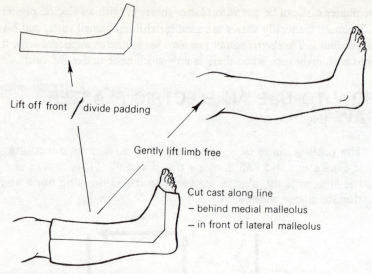

Lift off front / divide padding

Gently lift limb free

Cut cast along line
– behind medial malleolus
– in front of lateral malleolus

Fig. 14.2 How to bi-valve a plaster cast.

— Cut the cast on both sides of the limb *(bivalve)*, with care.
— Remove the front half of the cast, divide the underlying padding, then carefully lift the limb out of the back half of the cast.
— Reapply the bivalved cast and secure the two halves of the cast to the limb with crêpe bandages, for transport to the Radiology Department.

PRE-OPERATIVE PREPARATION OF A LIMB IMMOBILISED IN A PLASTER CAST

It may be necessary to operate upon a limb which has been immobilised for some weeks in a plaster cast. Before operation, the skin should be prepared to remove the dead superficial epidermis and hair. After a few weeks a fractured limb can be moved painlessly with gentleness and care.

PROCEDURE

— Bivalve the cast as described above.
— Gently remove the limb from the cast and place it on a sheet of polythene covered with a towel.
— Gently wash the limb with soap and water, if necessary using a soft nail brush, to remove the scaly skin.
— Shave the limb as necessary.
— Wrap the limb in a sterile towel and replace it in the bivalved cast.
— Apply a crêpe bandage or lengths of zinc oxide strapping to hold the cast together.

CUTTING A WINDOW IN A PLASTER CAST

It is sometimes necessary to expose a limited area of skin surface for examination, when it is inadvisable to remove or bivalve the whole cast. This can be achieved by cutting a window in the cast.

When it is known that a window will be cut later in a cast, for example for the removal of sutures, the site of the window can be indicated by applying additional dressings or a pad of wool over the wound, so that an elevation in the cast is produced.

HOW TO REMOVE WINDOW (Fig. 14.3)

— Identify and mark out on the cast the area of skin to be exposed, allowing a reasonable margin for error.
— Cut along the marks with an electric plaster saw.
— Gently lever the window out.
— Remove the underlying padding to expose the skin.

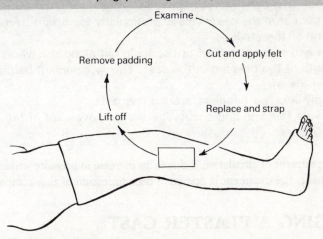

Fig. 14.3 Cutting a window in a plaster cast.

HOW TO REPLACE A WINDOW

The window must be replaced after examination, otherwise, if the limb swells, the skin will impinge against the cut edges of the cast and pressure sores will result. In addition the cast will be weakened.
— Remove any padding from the undersurface of the window.
— Cut a piece of orthopaedic felt to the exact size of the window, and stick it onto the undersurface of the window.
— Replace the window.
— Firmly apply zinc oxide strapping or plaster bandage around the cast to retain the window in position.

SPLITTING A PLASTER CAST

HOW TO SPLIT A PLASTER CAST

- *Make a longitudinal cut through the cast from one end to the other,* using plaster shears or an electric plaster saw.
  Note: It is useless and dangerous to nibble at the free edge of the cast under the misunderstanding that the swelling of the fingers or toes is due to constriction by the free edge of the cast. The swelling of the fingers or toes is indicative of increased pressure within the whole cast.
- Ease open the cut in the cast about $\frac{1}{4}$ to $\frac{1}{2}$ inch (0.6 to 1.25 cm).
- *Divide all padding including any wound dressings to expose the underlying skin.* Wound dressings must be cut as a blood-soaked gauze dressing dries rock hard and may itself form a constricting ring.
- *Check that bare skin is exposed throughout the whole length of the cut in the cast.* This is particularly important over the front of the ankle.
- Cut and place a strip of orthopaedic felt along the whole length of the opening in the cast. This will prevent herniation of the skin.
- Apply a crêpe bandage around the cast.
- *Elevate the limb and encourage active movement of the toes or fingers.*

When impairment of circulation is due to an increase in pressure within a fascial compartment, the treatment is operative decompression of that compartment.

WEDGING A PLASTER CAST

The aim when reducing a fracture is to reduce overlap and to obtain correct apposition and alignment of the fragments without rotation at the fracture site. It is difficult to maintain reduction during the application of a plaster cast. Post-reduction radiographs may show that although length and apposition have been satisfactorily obtained and rotation corrected, angulation at the fracture site is present. This can be corrected by wedging the plaster cast.

Charnley (1970) states that wedging of plaster casts should be regarded as an unfortunate necessity rather than a procedure of choice.

A wedge may be of the opening or closing type. In practice an opening wedge is preferable (Watson Jones, 1932). Charnley (1970) states that he has the impression that there is a higher incidence of delayed union when an opening wedge is used. He advises that wedging should be completed within the first 2 to 3 days after the application of the first plaster cast. If however wedging is delayed until the fracture is 'sticky', distraction of the fracture and delayed union are less likely to occur. *Only wedge a padded plaster cast.*

HOW TO WEDGE A PLASTER CAST (Fig. 14.4)

— Study the antero-posterior and lateral radiographs to determine in which direction angulation has occurred.
— Identify the level of the fracture. This can be done by comparing the radiographs with the cast, or more accurately by taking a radiograph after attaching a radio-opaque marker to the cast.

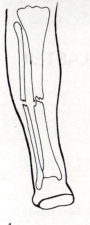 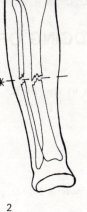 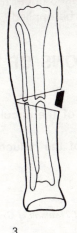 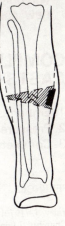

1
Study radiographs.
Check direction
of angulation.

2
Identify level and
site of hinge.
Mark cast.

3
Cut along mark.
Open wedge.
Insert wood
block.

4
Check radiograph.
Insert felt.
Replaster cast.

Fig. 14.4 Wedging a plaster cast. Note that in the above diagrams, angulation is shown on the antero-posterior radiograph only. If angulation is present on both the antero-posterior and the lateral radiographs, the apex of the wedge will be antero-medial/lateral or postero-medial/lateral, and the hinge must therefore be left at that site.

— Make a circumferential mark on the cast at the level of the fracture.
— Determine where on this mark the hinge of the wedge is to be located. The hinge is situated over the apex of the angulation when an opening wedge is proposed.
— Cut round the mark with an electric plaster saw, leaving 2 inches (5.0 cm) or one quarter of the circumference uncut, the site of the hinge.
— Slowly apply a corrective force to reduce the angulation, thus opening the wedge, the cast hinging on the uncut portion.
— Insert a wooden block to keep the wedge open. Temporarily secure the block with zinc oxide strapping.
— Take radiographs to determine whether adequate correction has been obtained. If not, open or close the wedge as required.

— If correction has been obtained, cut and insert a strip of orthopaedic felt the size of the wedge, *leaving the wooden block in place.*
— Apply plaster bandages around the cast.
— *Change the plaster cast*
    1. If pain persists for more than 1 to 2 hours after wedging.
    2. *Routinely two weeks after wedging.* Any plaster cast can only be wedged once. If more correction is required, a new cast must be applied.

COMPLICATIONS OF WEDGING OF PLASTER CASTS

1. Embarrassment of the circulation in the limb.
2. Pressure sores.
3. Complete loss of the reduction.

REFERENCES

Charnley, J. (1970) *The Closed Treatment of Common Fractures,* 3rd edn, p. 231. Edinburgh: Churchill Livingstone.
English, M. (1957) *Plaster-of-Paris Technique.* Edinburgh: E. & S. Livingstone.
Powell, M. (1968) *Orthopaedic Nursing,* 6th edn. Edinburgh: E. & S. Livingstone.
Smith & Nephew Ltd *Gypsona Technique,* 16th edn. Welwyn Garden City, Herts.
Watson-Jones, R. (1932) The treatment of fractures of the shafts of the tibia and fibula. *Journal of Bone and Joint Surgery,* **14,** 591.

15.

Functional bracing

Functional bracing is a closed method of treating fractures based on the belief that continuing function, while a fracture is uniting, encourages osteogenesis, promotes the healing of tissues and prevents the development of joint stiffness, thus accelerating rehabilitation. The concept accepts that the loss of the anatomical reduction of a fracture is a small price to pay for rapid healing and the restoration of function, without compromising the appearance of the limb by operative scars (Sarmiento and Latta, 1981). It complements rather than replaces other forms of treatment.

The concept of functional bracing is not new. In 1855 H.H. Smith, a surgeon in Philadelphia, designed an appliance for the ambulant treatment of cases of non-union of the proximal femur. It consisted of a waist band, ischial support and a thigh-lacer, as well as knee and ankle hinges. Union occurred in the seven patients treated. In this century, Lucas-Championnière (1910) advocated early weight-bearing for tibial fractures treated in plaster casts, believing that 'Life is Motion'. In 1926, Gurd (1940) recommended immediate weight-bearing in an unpadded below-knee cast, of the pattern later used by Sarmiento, for fractures of the ankle and foot.

The present era of functional bracing probably began during the 1950s when Dehne used this method for the treatment of fractures of the shaft of the tibia in American troops (Dehne et al, 1961). Mooney et al (1970) stated that one thousand cases were treated. Non-union and persistent infection did not occur despite an approximate incidence of compound fractures of thirty per cent. In 1963, Sarmiento began his systematic study of functional bracing with both basic and clinical research.

THE THEORETICAL BASIS OF FUNCTIONAL BRACING

Fractured ribs unite. This indicates that the elimination of movement at a fracture site is not mandatory for a fracture to unite. It is stability that is important, to reduce pain, maintain alignment and prevent deformity.

If the fragments of a fracture are held rigidly together, the formation of external bridging callus is suppressed (Anderson, 1965) and union occurs by the formation of medullary callus. If some movement occurs between the fragments, external bridging callus forms, and as it is situated at a distance from the axis of potential movement, it has a greater mechanical advantage than medullary callus, and therefore makes a much stronger early repair. Sarmiento asserts that rigid immobilisation is detrimental to fracture healing and that the intermittent loading of the fracture area, by muscle activity and weight bearing, promotes local blood flow and the development of electrical fields which are beneficial for healing.

A fracture brace which allows movement at the joints and some movement at the fracture site transmits a measurable load which decreases as the fracture progresses to union (Meggitt et al, 1981; Wardlaw et al, 1981). In the early stages of union it is the soft tissue mass that transmits most of the load. The muscle compartments act as a fluid mass surrounded by an elastic container, the deep fascia. Fluid is not compressible and the fascia cannot be stretched beyond the confines of the cast. In this way, after a certain degree of displacement, pressure and load is transmitted without further deformation (Fig. 15.1). Elastic recoil takes place when the load is reduced. When muscles contract, they bulge. When

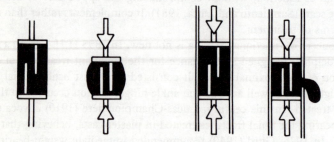

Fig. 15.1 Diagramatic illustration of how load is transmitted by muscle within a rigid container (the cast) as long as the fascia is intact (after Sarmiento & Latta, 1981).

this occurs within a rigid constraining cylinder, the muscles are forced inwards away from the rigid walls and against the central fragments thus causing the bony fragments to be held more firmly (Fig. 15.2).

Soft tissues are excellent at resisting tension as long as they have not been damaged too severely by the injury. The hydraulic forces described above control the fragments and resist overlap and angulation until callus forms and takes over that function. Rotation is resisted usually by components of the brace and/or the tendency of muscle contraction and joint movement to align the fragments.

Sarmiento and Latta (1981) have shown that in closed fractures, shortening does not increase with weight-bearing, although the original amount of shortening does persist. In tibial fractures they found this to be only $\frac{1}{4}-\frac{3}{8}$ inches (6.0–9.0 mm). In compound fractures, or others where there is a severe disruption of the soft tissues, there is insufficient tissue linking the fragments of bone to resist overlap, despite the hydraulic forces which also act. These

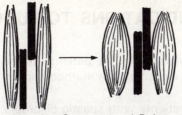

Muscles Contract and Bulge
Increased Overlap of Fracture

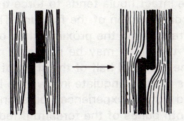

When Muscles Contract Within Rigid
Cylinder They do not Bulge. Bony
Fragments Held More Firmly.

Fig. 15.2   When muscles contract within a rigid cylinder they are forced inwards away from the rigid walls thus holding the bony fragments more firmly.

fractures will shorten excessively if weight-bearing is allowed before the soft tissues have healed. An initial period of conventional treatment is therefore essential with such fractures.

WHEN TO APPLY A FUNCTIONAL BRACE

Functional braces usually are not applied at the time of injury. Conventional casts, which immobilise the joints above and below the fracture, or traction may be used initially, care being taken during this time to correct any angular or rotational deformity as the position following the cast bracing of a fracture is basically dependent upon the position of the fragments before the brace is applied. Compound fractures will not be ready for bracing as soon as closed fractures.

Assess the fracture clinically when pain and swelling have subsided.

1. Minor movements at the fracture site should be painless.
2. Any deformity should disappear once the deforming force is removed.
3. There should be reasonable resistance to telescoping.
4. Shortening should not excede $\frac{1}{4}$ inch (6.0 mm) for the tibia and $\frac{1}{2}$ inch (1.25 cm) for the femur.

CONTRA-INDICATIONS TO FUNCTIONAL BRACING

1. Lack of co-operation by the patient. As the co-operation of the patient is essential, the method cannot be used if this is uncertain.
2. Fractures in patients with spastic disorders, as there is a tendency for the fractures to angulate within the brace.
3. Deficient sensibility of the limb.
4. When a brace cannot be fitted closely and accurately, as a close fit with the minimum of padding is essential.
5. Isolated fractures of the tibia. These should be treated with caution, as the intact fibula tends to force the limb into varus and to delay consolidation of the fracture. This is more marked with fractures in the proximal third of the tibia. Osteotomy of the fibula may be needed.
6. Fractures in the proximal half of the shaft of the femur. As these fractures tend to angulate into varus, bracing should only be carried out by experienced personnel.
7. Fractures of both bones of the forearm if reduction has been difficult.
8. Isolated fractures of the radius with damage to the inferior radio-ulnar joint or interosseous membrane.
9. Isolated fractures of the ulna with damage to the superior radio-ulnar joint.

THE USE OF MODERN MATERIALS IN FUNCTIONAL BRACING

Many of the modern synthetic casting materials are well-suited for use in the functional bracing of fractures (see p. 196). Those supplied in the form of bandages are light and strong, and are used in the same way as plaster-of-Paris. Many of them are sufficiently flexible to allow the brace to be loosened and tightened after it has been split longitudinally and straps attached.

Thermoplastic casting materials supplied in sheets, such as Orthoplast (Johnson & Johnson Ltd)* and Hexcelite (Orthopaedic Systems)* require a different technique, involving the careful use of patterns, before the final shape is cut from a large and expensive sheet of material. Kits are available commercially (Johnson & Johnson Ltd). Braces made from thermoplastic material are easily modified by local heating of the area to be altered.

Prefabricated plastic femoral and tibial braces are available (United States Manufacturing Co.)* in a range of sizes. Fitting of these should be straight-forward as long as the limb conforms to one of the standard shapes, and attention is paid to preventing excessive pressure on the skin at the knee and ankle.

*See Appendix.

FUNCTIONAL BRACING FOR FRACTURES OF THE TIBIA

Sarmiento and Latta (1981) found that external bridging callus did not form satisfactorily in response to the functional bracing of tibial fractures, unless the brace was applied within six weeks of the fracture occurring. After this time there was a higher incidence of delayed and non-union.

For fractures of the tibial plateau, a cast brace incorporating hinges is required.

HOW TO APPLY A FUNCTIONAL BRACE FOR THE TIBIA

1. Using plaster-of-Paris: the Sarmiento tibial plaster cast (Fig. 15.3)

— Remove the original cast and any transfixing pins, and cover any pin holes with small dry dressings.
— Sit the patient on a couch with his legs dangling over the edge and the relevant thigh supported on a sand bag. Encourage the patient to relax.
— Liberally dust the leg with non-perfumed talcum powder, before rolling the cast sock or stockinette onto the limb from the toes to above the knee, taking care to avoid any wrinkles.
— Apply minimal orthopaedic wool padding over the heel, tendo calcaneus, malleoli, common peroneal nerve and tibial condyles and crest.

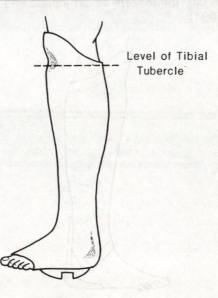

Level of Tibial
Tubercle

Fig. 15.3 The Sarmiento tibial plaster cast.

— With the ankle at a right angle, apply plaster-of-Paris bandages from the toes to 2 inches (5.0 cm) above the ankle, moulding carefully around the ankle.

— Apply further plaster-of-Paris from the toes to the tibial tuberosity and mould it over the medial proximal half of the soft tissues of the calf, aiming to reproduce the shape of the sound leg.

— Flex the knee to 40 degrees and rest the patient's heel on your lap.

— Apply further plaster-of-Paris from the top of the cast to 1 inch (2.5 cm) above the proximal pole of the patella.

— Firmly mould the plaster cast over the medial flare of the tibia and the patellar tendon. At the same time apply firm pressure in the popliteal fossa and the back of the calf with the flat of the hand, to produce a triangular cross-section in this area to help to control rotation.

— Mark out and trim the upper end of the cast, keeping the ears as long as possible on both sides of the knee. Posteriorly the upper edge of the cast is level with the tibial tuberosity. Inferiorly the toes must be free to flex and extend fully (Fig. 15.3).

— Fit a walking heel slightly anteriorly to the long axis of the tibia.

2. Using thermoplastic material (Orthoplast) (Fig. 15.4)

This account is based on the instruction sheet from Johnson & Johnson Ltd, the makers of Orthoplast and a paper by Suman (1981).

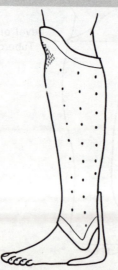

Fig. 15.4 Orthoplast tibial functional brace.

Two people are required. The patient must be able to co-operate without sedation.

— Remove the original cast and any transifixing pins, and cover any pin holes with small dry dressings.
— Sit the patient on a couch with his legs dangling over the edge and the relevant thigh supported on a sand bag. Encourage the patient to relax.
— Roll a double layer of stockinette onto the limb from the middle of the foot to above the knee, taking care to avoid any wrinkles.
— Wrap a layer of adhesive foam around the ankle to protect the malleoli, and one or two layers of orthopaedic wool padding, if necessary, over the tibial crest and condyles.
— Cut a pattern from thin card (Fig. 15.5) and trim it so that it extends from the middle of the patella to the tips of the malleoli. It should wrap around the shin and overlap by 2 inches (5.0 cm) in the mid-line posteriorly. If a tibial bracing kit is being used, choose and trim the most suitable of the three half patterns supplied in the kit.

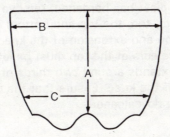

Fig. 15.5 Shape of pattern for Orthoplast tibial functional brace. A. Distance from superior pole of patella to ankle joint. B. Circumference at level of tibial condyles, plus 2 inches (5.0 cm). C. Circumference around ankle at level of malleoli, plus 2 inches (5.0 cm).

— Mark out the final shape on the sheet of perforated Orthoplast.
— Check with a tape measure (Fig. 15.5) that A, the mid-anterior vertical line of the marked shape is equal to the distance from the top of the patella to the inter-malleolar line; B, the width at the level of the tibial condyles is equal to the circumference there plus 2 inches (5.0 cm); and C, the width 1 inch (2.5 cm) above the malleoli is equal to the circumference there plus 2 inches (5.0 cm).
— Cut the Orthoplast sheet as marked, heat it in a water bath at a temperature of 72 to 77°C for three minutes, and then dab it dry.

— Support the patient's leg with the knee flexed about 40 degrees by resting the heel on your knee.
— While holding the edges apart at the back mould the supple sheet of Orthoplast over the leg until the front is perfectly smooth and contoured. Then temporarily bond the sheet to itself by pinching the pieces together posteriorly to form a vertical seam. This enables a snug fit to be made all the way down.
— Trim the protruding layers to a width of 1 inch (2.5 cm), degrease the surfaces which are to be bonded, with trichloroethane or carbon tetrachloride and then fold down the seam so that it lies flat.
— Firmly wrap a cold, wet elasticated bandage over the brace from the ankle to the knee to assist close moulding and accelerate setting.
— As soon as the wet bandage has been applied firmly, mould the Orthoplast on either side of the tibial crest to provide a relief channel (Fig. 15.6), over the patellar tendon to ensure that the brace is patellar tendon bearing, and in the politeal fossa to produce a triangular cross section in this area to help to control rotation.
— When the Orthoplast has hardened, remove the wet bandage and with scissors, trim the top and bottom edges of the brace. Full flexion and extension of the knee must be possible, and the ears at the top must be left long enough so that the brace extends around two thirds of the circumference of the knee. Ensure that the brace does not press on the tendo calcaneus.

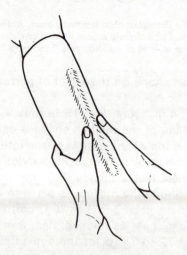

Fig. 15.6 Moulding Orthoplast on both sides of tibial crest to provide a relief channel.

— Fold the stockinette over the edges of the Orthoplast and
secure with adhesive tape (Fig. 15.4).
— Fit a heel cup (see below).

HEEL-CUPS

The purpose of a heel-cup is to help to control rotation and to stop the brace
sliding down the leg. It will also give some lateral support.

1. A simple form of heel-cup can be made from a strip of plain Orthoplast
measuring 11 by 3 inches (27.0 by 7.5 cm). After the usual heating, drying and
degreasing, attach the strip to the back of the brace so that it covers the back of
the ankle and heel and then extends forwards under the heel to the front of the os
calcis (Fig. 15.4).

2. Ready-moulded polypropylene heel-cups are available (Fig. 15.7). Choose
the appropriate size of heel-cup and secure it to the lower end of the brace by
wrapping a strip of Orthoplast, measuring approximately 9 by 4 inches (23.0 by
10.0 cm) over the uprights of the heel-cup, after the usual heating, drying and
degreasing.

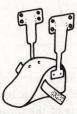

Fig. 15.7   Ready-moulded polypropylene heel-cup.

Once the heel-cup is attached, the patient should be able to wear ordinary
shoes and walk with a normal gait. In addition, the heel-cup can be swung
backwards to allow the patient to wash the foot and to put on a sock under the
heel-cup.

Excoriation of the skin under a thermoplastic brace can occur due to excessive
sweating. This problem can be overcome by making the brace removable. To do
this, the brace is split from top to bottom posteriorly, using short even vertical
strokes with a cast cutting saw. Care is essential to avoid overheating and the
possibility of burning the patient's skin. Velcro straps are then fitted.

FUNCTIONAL BRACING FOR FRACTURES OF
THE FEMUR

Many authors (Mooney et al, 1970; Connolly et al, 1973) state that long-leg cast
braces should only be used in the management of fractures in the distal half of
the shaft of the femur, as these braces cannot control the tendency of fractures in
the proximal third of the femur to go into varus, from the pull of the hip

abductor and adductor muscles. To control fractures in the proximal third of the femur, this tendency to varus angulation must be resisted. This requires the thigh cast to be attached proximally to a pelvic band via a hip joint.

Meggitt et al (1981) have designed a hip-hinge thigh-cast brace (Fig. 15.8) for use in the management of this fracture. The thigh-cast, quadrilateral in shape to

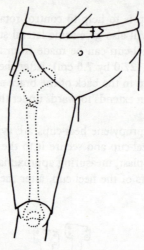

Fig. 15.8 Hip-hinge thigh cast brace.

resist torsion, extends distally to just above the knee. Proximally it is attached by a metal uniplanar hip hinge to a rigid pelvic band, fitted with an adjustable waist belt and shoulder strap. The axis of the hinge is set level with the tip of the greater trochanter in a position of 20 degrees of abduction at the hip. In 24 patients with fractures of the proximal half of the shaft of the femur, union occurred after between 11 and 18 weeks, and varus angulation was not a problem.

In fractures of the distal two thirds of the shaft of the femur Meggitt et al (1981) claim that a long-leg cast brace functions mainly as an anti-buckling hinged tube. They feel that once telescoping of the fracture has ceased, the fracture receives little hydraulic support from the muscles, being supported instead, by the thigh-cast, knee hinges and upper shin cast which transmits between 10 and 30% of body weight. The ankle and foot section of the brace immobilises the foot, ankle and calf and only acts as a static support for that part of the brace above. They suggest therefore, that a standard long-leg cast brace should be used only for the management of fractures of the distal half of the shaft of the femur and of the tibial plateau, in obese patients with flabby thighs and without a waist. For these fractures in patients who are not obese and who have a more muscular and cylindrical shaped thigh, they suggest a knee-hinge cylinder cast brace suspended from a waist band (Fig. 15.9). A similar reduced femoral cast brace is described by Sarmiento and Latta (1981), the brace below the knee being reduced to an encircling calf band, with the lower arms of the metal knee hinges being riveted to a plastic heel-cup (Fig. 15.10).

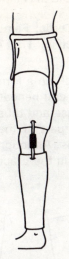

Fig. 15.9 Knee-hinge cylinder cast brace, using metal knee hinges.

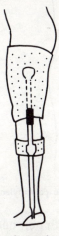

Fig. 15.10 Femoral functional brace in thermoplastic material.

HOW TO APPLY A LONG LEG CAST BRACE

This type of cast brace (Fig. 15.11) is used for the treatment of fractures of the distal half of the shaft of the femur and of the tibial plateau. Full extension of the knee and sufficient callus to prevent shortening must be present, and pain and marked mobility at the fracture site must be absent. Most fractures can be braced within four to six weeks of injury.

Various types of plaster or thermoplastic materials may be used. The brace is constructed in four separate stages: general preparation, below-knee cast, thigh cast and fitting of knee hinges.

1. Using Orthoflex and Zoroc: Femoral Functional Bracing Kit
(Johnson & Johnson Ltd) (Fig. 15.11)

a. *General preparation*
— Sit the patient on a couch on a firm pad to ensure clearance
   of about 6 inches (15.0 cm) beneath the patient's thigh. This
   exposes the gluteal crease and thus allows the smooth
   application of the thigh part of the brace.
— Remove any traction pins. Although traction pins can be left
   in situ and incorporated in the brace, application is easier if
   they are removed.

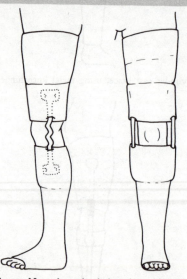

Fig. 15.11 Long leg cast brace. Note the polyethylene knee hinges.

— Liberally dust the limb with non-perfumed talcum powder, to
   make the application of the cast sock or stockinette easier.
— Roll the cast sock onto the limb from the toes to the groin
   taking care to avoid wrinkles, and ask the patient to hold the
   cast sock high into the groin and gluteal crease all the time.
— Apply minimal orthopaedic wool padding over the heel, tendo
   calcaneus, malleoli, tibial crest and condyles and the common
   peroneal nerve.
— With the adhesive surface facing outwards to prevent
   possible skin reaction apply a pre-cut piece of orthopaedic
   felt over the tibial condyles, making sure that the double layer
   is on the medial side to assist in the alignment of the hinges
   (Fig. 15.12).
— Apply a second pre-cut piece of orthopaedic felt over the
   femoral condyles again with the adhesive surface facing
   outwards, but with the double layer on the lateral side (Fig.
   15.12).

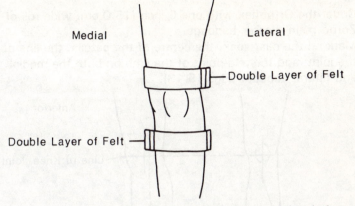

Fig. 15.12 To show how the orthopaedic felt is applied above and below the knee.

b. *Below-knee cast*
— With the ankle at a right angle, apply one 5 inch (12.5 cm) wide roll of Orthoflex elastic plaster bandage from the base of the toes to within $\frac{1}{4}$ inch (6.0 mm) of the top of the orthopaedic felt. The bandage must be rolled on and NOT tensioned, to avoid an unduly tight cast.
— Cover the Orthoflex with one 6 inch (15.0 cm) wide roll of Zoroc resin plaster bandage.
— Carefully mould the cast around the heel and ankle and wait until it sets.

c. *Thigh cast*
— Support the leg and exert slight traction on the limb maintaining the correct rotational position.
— Make sure that the cast sock is held high up into the groin and gluteal crease.
— Heat the pre-cut Orthoplast cast brim in a water bath at a temperature of 72–77°C for three minutes, mop off the surface water and fit the cast brim snugly around the upper thigh ensuring a close fit at the groin.
— Trim and smooth the upper edges of the cast brim. This is helped by firmly pulling the cast sock down over the upper edge of the Orthoplast.
— Apply a cold wet elasticated bandage over the Orthoplast.
— Mould the cast brim into a quadrilateral shape by applying pressure with both hands. Maintain this pressure until the Orthoplast hardens. The quadrilateral shape of the upper part of the thigh cast helps to control rotation.
— Firmly apply one 5 inch (12.5 cm) wide roll of Orthoflex elastic plaster bandage around the thigh from $\frac{1}{4}$ inch (6.0 mm) above the lower edge of the orthopaedic felt to $\frac{1}{2}$ inch (1.25 cm) below the top of the cast brim. Do not apply the Orthoflex under tension.

— Cover the Orthoflex with one 6 inch (15.0 cm) wide roll of Zoroc resin plaster bandage.
— Mark on the cast sock, the centre of the patella, the line of the joint, and the mid-point of the limb on both the medial and lateral aspects (Fig. 15.13).

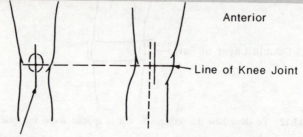

Anterior

Line of Knee Joint

Centre of Patella   Line for Knee Hinges

Fig. 15.13 Mark on the cast sock, the centre of the patella, the line of the knee joint, and the mid-point of the limb on both sides. The hatched line indicates the position for the knee hinges.

d. *Hinges*

These may be of polyethylene (as supplied in the kit), or metal. Metal hinges must be positioned accurately using a jig. Accurate positioning of the polyethylene hinges is not so important as they do not have a localised axis of rotation. In addition their side arms cannot be shaped to fit the contours of the limb.

(i) *Polyethylene hinges* (Fig. 15.14)

— Make a slab from one half of a 6 inch (15.0 cm) wide Zoroc bandage and place it over the front of the lower part of the thigh cast.
— Position the hinges on the slab so that they lie just behind the mid-point of the limb on each side of the knee (Fig. 15.13). Fold back the ends of the slab over the ends of the hinges and then, using the remains of the above Zoroc bandage, firmly bind the hinges to the thigh cast by twisting the bandage into a rope as it crosses the hinges. The hinges are covered completely from the corrugated section to the top.

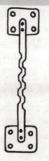

Fig. 15.14 Polyethylene knee hinge.

— Wait until the above plaster is set and then make another slab
  from a similar roll of Zoroc bandage and place it over the
  upper margin of the below-knee part of the brace.
— While maintaining traction on the limb, push the thigh cast
  proximally and then bind the lower part of the hinges to the
  below-knee part of the cast in an identical manner as before.
— Turn the cast sock back over the lower end of the brace at
  the toes and fix it in position with a 4 inch (10.0 cm) wide
  roll of Zoroc bandage using the rest of the bandage to
  reinforce the sole of the brace.
— After the plaster has set, ask the patient to gently flex the
  knee. Trim the brace as necessary to ensure that it is
  comfortable and that flexion of the knee to 90 degrees is not
  impeded.
— After 24 hours, give the patient a plaster boot and allow him
  to begin mobilising, taking as much weight through the
  brace, as he can.

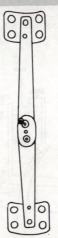

Fig. 15.15   Metal knee hinge.

(ii) *Metal hinges* (Fig. 15.15)
— Temporarily lock the metal hinges in extension and then fit
  them to the jig, to hold them parallel (Fig. 15.16).

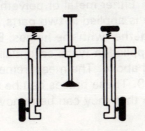
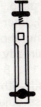

Fig. 15.16   Jig to hold the metal knee hinges parallel.

- Offer up the hinges in the jig to the limb and hold them at the level of the middle of the patella and about $\frac{3}{4}$ inch (2.0 cm) behind the mid-point of the limb on each side.
- Shape the arms of the hinges with bending irons, so that the plates at the end of the arms rest snugly against the cast.
- Check that the hinges are orientated correctly to allow flexion of the knee and do not rub on the sides of the limb.
- Clamp the lower ends of the hinges to the below-knee cast with a giant jubilee clip.
- While maintaining traction on the limb, push the thigh cast proximally and then clamp the upper ends of the hinges to the thigh cast with a second jubilee clip. This will seat the thigh cast as firmly as possible.
- With the jubilee clips in position (Fig. 15.17), plaster the ends of the hinges onto the casts above and below the clips, then remove the clips and complete the attachment of the hinges.
- Remove the jig and the locking screws from the hinges, and check that the axis of movement looks correct when the knee is flexed gently, as far as the patient will tolerate.
- Finish off the lower end of the brace and trim it as described above.

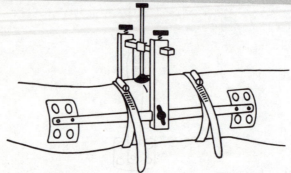

Fig. 15.17 Jig holding metal knee hinges in position with pointer over the centre of the patella, and giant jubilee clips holding arms of hinges to the cast.

2. Using thermoplastic material

A functional brace for the femur can be made from thermoplastic materials. Either metal or polyethylene hinges can be used. The brace is applied in two parts, tibial and femoral, later joined together with the hinges. Both the tibial and femoral parts are applied in ways essentially identical to those already described above. The measurements are shown in Figs 15.18 and 15.19. These braces can be split and fastened with straps so that they can be removed or their tightness adjusted.

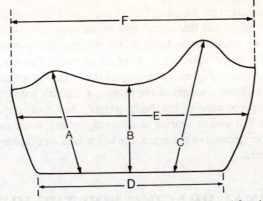

Fig. 15.18 Shape of pattern for Orthoplast for femoral part of femoral functional brace. A. Distance from ischial tuberosity to medial femoral condyle. B. Distance from groin to medial femoral condyle. C. Distance from tip of greater trochanter to lateral femoral condyle. D. Circumference of thigh at level of femoral condyles plus 1 inch (2.5 cm). E. Circumference at mid-thigh plus 1 inch (2.5 cm). F. Oblique circumference at groin plus 1 inch (2.5 cm).

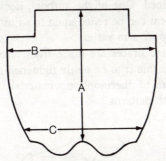

Fig. 15.19 Shape of pattern for Orthoplast for tibial part of femoral functional brace. A. Distance from tibial plateau to ankle joint plus 1 inch (2.5 cm). B. Circumference at level of tibial condyles plus 1 inch (2.5 cm). C. Circumference around ankle at level of malleoli plus 1 inch (2.5 cm).

WHEN TO DISCARD A FEMORAL CAST BRACE

Mooney et al (1970) determined empirically to remove a femoral cast brace on the basis of the function and not the radiological appearance of the injured limb. They felt that what was important was that the patient could use the limb without distress, could tolerate full weight bearing and had sufficient active use of the knee for walking and sitting.

It has been shown (Meggitt et al, 1981; Wardlaw et al, 1981) in studies of fractures of the distal two thirds of the shaft of the femur using strain gauges incorporated into long-leg cast braces, that the thigh section of the cast brace carries on average 10–30% of the weight of the body, during healing of the fracture. As the fracture progresses towards union, the percentage of the weight of the body transmitted by the limb increases until full weight bearing occurs. From these observations Meggitt et al (1981) developed a crude but simple and practical test, using bathroom scales, to determine when it is safe to remove the brace.

The patient stands erect with the foot of the braced limb on bathroom scales and the foot of the normal limb supported at the same level on wooden blocks. Using a frame or crutches for balance, the patient slowly transfers as much weight as possible to the fractured limb for ten seconds. This is repeated several times until a consistent highest recording of the 'standing weight' is obtained. From this and the known weight of the patient, a 'fracture load-bearing index' is calculated as a percentage of the body weight. As union occurs, this index increases. When full weight bearing is achieved, the cast brace can be removed. Immediately after removal of the brace, the index falls, but rapidly recovers after one to three weeks.

FUNCTIONAL BRACING FOR THE HUMERUS
(Fig. 15.20)

Sarmiento and Latta (1981) do not advise bracing for ten to fifteen days after the fracture has been sustained. One of the authors, however, will apply a brace much earlier, if the patient can be relied upon to adjust the tension of the brace as the swelling of the upper arm varies.

It is essential that these braces are made from material which is light and sufficiently flexible to enable it to be easily tightened and loosened around the upper arm. Thin sheets of thermoplastic material, such as Orthoplast are available in kit form with patterns.

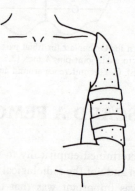

Fig. 15.20 Functional brace for the humerus.

HOW TO APPLY A FUNCTIONAL BRACE FOR THE HUMERUS

— Give adequate analgesia to allow the injured arm to be moved a little.
— Sit the patient on a chair with the injured upper limb supported by a collar and cuff, with the elbow at a right angle.

— Draw on the arm an outline of where the brace is to lie, or if a commercial kit is being used, choose the pattern of the correct size (Fig. 15.21). The brace must be free of the elbow crease and the axilla, but must extend almost to the olecranon and the point of the shoulder. It must not extend beyond the elbow or shoulder as this will restrict subsequent movement (Fig. 15.20).

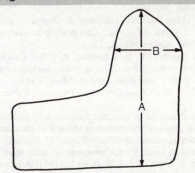

Fig. 15.21 Shape of pattern for Orthoplast functional brace for the humerus. A. Distance from 3 inches (7.5 cm) above the shoulder joint to the inner crease of the elbow. B. Circumference of upper arm at the level of the axilla plus 2 inches (5.0 cm).

— Cut a sheet of Orthoplast to conform to the outline on the upper arm or to the pattern, allowing a generous overlap.
— Ask the patient to lean towards the injured side, to allow the upper arm to hang free of the side of the chest.
— Apply a cast sock or a double layer of stockinette over the upper arm.
— Heat the Orthoplast in a water bath at a temperature of 72 to 77°C for three minutes, dab it dry, sprinkle talcum powder where the material will overlap to prevent it from self-bonding, and then shape the supple material around the upper arm. It may be more convenient to carry out the initial rough moulding on the patient's sound upper limb.
— Wrap a cold wet elasticated bandage over the Orthoplast.
— When the Orthoplast has hardened, remove the wet bandage and then the brace and trim the brace until it fits comfortably and all its edges are smooth.
— Attach Velcro straps and check that the patient can manipulate them.
— Turn the cast sock or stockinette over the upper and lower edges of the brace and secure it with adhesive tape.
— Tell the patient that the brace must always be kept wrapped as firmly as possible around the limb, consistent with comfort.
— Show the patient how to remove the collar and cuff, flex and extend the elbow, and carry out pendulum movements of the shoulder.

REFERENCES

Anderson, L.D. (1965) Compression plate fixation and the effect of different types of internal fixation on fracture healing. *Journal of Bone and Joint Surgery,* **47-A,** 191.

Connolly, J.F., Dehne, E. & Lafollette, B. (1973) Closed reduction and early cast-brace ambulation in the treatment of femoral fractures. Part II: Results in one hundred and forty-three fractures. *Journal of Bone and Joint Surgery,* **55-A,** 1581.

Dehne, E., Metz, C.W., Deffer, P.A. & Hall, R.M. (1961) Non-operative treatment of the fractured tibia by immediate weight-bearing. *Journal of Trauma,* **2,** 514.

Gurd, F.B. (1940) The ambulatory treatment of fractures of the lower extremity. *Surgery, Gynaecology and Obstetrics,* **70,** 385.

Lucas-Championnière, J. (1910) *Precis du Traitment des Fractures,* p. 64. Paris: Steinheil.

Meggitt, B.F., Juett, D.A. & Smith, J.D. (1981) Cast-bracing for fractures of the femoral shaft. *Journal of Bone and Joint Surgery,* **63-B,** 12.

Mooney, V., Nickel, V.L., Harvey, J.P. Jr. & Snelson, R. (1970) Cast-brace treatment for fractures of the distal part of the femur. A prospective controlled study of one hundred and fifty patients. *Journal of Bone and Joint Surgery,* **52-A,** 1563.

Sarmiento, A. & Latta, L.L. (1981) *Closed Functional Treatment of Fractures.* Berlin: Springer-Verlag.

Smith, H.H. (1855) On the treatment of ununited fractures by means of artificial limbs, which combine the principle of pressure and motion at the seat of the fracture and lead to the formation of an ensheathing callus. *American Journal of Medical Science,* **29,** 102.

Suman, R.K. (1981) Orthoplast brace for the treatment of tibial shaft fractures. *Inury,* **13,** 133.

Wardlaw, D., McLaughlan, J., Pratt, D.J. & Bowker, P. (1981) A biomechanical study of cast-brace treatment of femoral shaft fractures. *Journal of Bone and Joint Surgery,* **63-B,** 7.

16.

External skeletal fixation

The term external skeletal fixation is used to describe the method whereby bones and bone fragments are held rigidly by metal pins, which transfix the individual bone fragments but not necessarily the limb, and which are themselves attached securely to a strong external frame. The main supporting frame is attached to the ends of the pins thus keeping it clear of the soft tissues and therefore leaving room for dressings or procedures such as skin grafting to be carried out. Foreign material is not placed at the site of intended bony union. Rigid fixation of the fracture minimises the risk of infection (Hicks, 1970). This method of 'immobilisation' of bone falls between plaster casts and internal fixation with plates and screws or nails.

DEVELOPMENT OF EXTERNAL FIXATION SYSTEMS

The concept of external fixation of fractures is not new. For many years it has been standard practice when a fracture of the femur is present, to immobilise a fracture of the ipsilateral tibia by transfixing it above and below the fracture site with Steinmann pins which are then incorporated in a plaster-of-Paris cast.

Charnley compression clamps are a form of external fixation which have been used for many years when performing an arthrodesis. The bone on each side of the joint is transfixed by a Steinmann pin. Simple clamps attach threaded connecting rods to the ends of the pins. When wing nuts on the connecting rods are turned, the Steinmann pins are approximated and the prepared bone ends are brought and held rigidly together under compression.

Various external fixation frames were developed to control the osteotomy site in leg-lengthening procedures. The earliest was probably that of Putti (Abbott, 1927), who in 1921 transfixed each half of the bone and soft tissue on both sides with a pin, and placed spring metal struts between the ends of the pins. Abbott developed the idea with two pins above and below the osteotomy site, to improve control of angulation. These frames were rarely used for treating fractures. In 1938, Hoffmann, a Swiss doctor, designed an external fixation system specifically for the treatment of fractures. This system was used until 1968, when the original concept was modified by Vidal in France. This work resulted in the construction of a frame which allowed for both the reduction of the fracture after assembly of the frame, as well as the provision of rigid stabilisation of the most severe fractures of long bones.

There are now several external fixation systems commercially available. They all follow the same basic principles.

THE PRINCIPLES OF EXTERNAL FIXATION SYSTEMS

PINS

Although only one pin may be placed in each site, it is more usual for two or three pins to be placed close together to obtain a firmer grip on the bone and to prevent rotation.

Transfixing pins

These pass through the bone and the soft tissues on both sides of the limb. Although a more secure grip on the bone and the frame will be obtained, they may cause damage to vital soft tissues. They are not recommended for use in the upper limb, or upper femur.

Transfixing pins may be completely smooth or have a centrally raised threaded section. They are available in different diameters and overall lengths and with threaded sections of various length to allow the correct size to be chosen for each patient. The correct transfixing pin is where the length of the threaded section is several threads longer than the diameter of the diaphysis or metaphysis into which it is to be inserted.

Half-pins

These do not pass through the whole limb. They are inserted from one side of the limb only, thus reducing the danger of damage to vital soft tissues. They must however pass through the whole width of the bone, penetrating both cortices. Generally they are used in the upper limb, pelvis and upper part of the thigh. Half-pins may be self-drilling and self-tapping and the threaded section may be continuous or interrupted.

Those half-pins with a continuous threaded section are used commonly in cancellous bone. The length of the threaded section should exceed the diameter of the bone by several threads. If a half-pin with a continuous threaded section is to be inserted into the diaphysis of a long bone, the bone must be drilled before the half-pin is inserted.

Half-pins with an interrupted thread are used primarily in long bones where a good purchase can be obtained in both cortices. If a self-drilling and tapping pin with a continuous thread is inserted into a diaphysis of a long bone, there is a danger that the thread, cut in the first cortex, will be damaged when the pin is being drilled through the second cortex. The use of a pin with an interrupted thread avoids this as the smooth central section of the shank will still be in the first cortex while the second cortex is being drilled. Once the second cortex has been perforated both sections of the thread will be screwed into their respective cortices (Fig. 16.1). A radiograph is needed to help choose the correct length of half-pins with an interrupted thread.

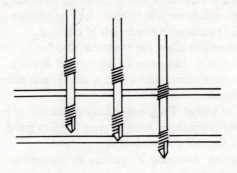

Fig. 16.1 If self-drilling and tapping pins are used, the threaded section must be interrupted, and the pins must be of the correct length.

FRAMES

Although in an emergency, frames can be constructed from different materials in a variety of ways, using for example plaster-of-Paris, Nissen U-loop or Charnley compression clamps, commercially available frames are better.

Many of the different types of frame use a variety of clamps, universal joints and rods of varying length to construct the frame. Some frames are more rigid than others. They also differ by the ease with which the frame is constructed and by which the position of the bony fragments can be adjusted, once the frame has been constructed. The more complex frames permit the correction of angulation and rotation as well as the distraction or compression of the bony fragments. With some frames, the pins in each group must be inserted parallel to one another for the clamps to fit, and therefore it is important to use a jig in their insertion. Other frames have clamps which can accommodate groups of pins which are not parallel to each other.

Some modern external fixation systems incorporate a layer of insulating material in the clamps to prevent electrolytic action if slightly dissimilar metals are used, and to prevent distortion of any electrical fields that may be added from internal or external electrodes separate from the frame.

After construction, some external fixation systems can be suspended from a Balkan beam, by attaching cords and weights. Elevation will help to reduce swelling, prevent compression of soft tissues, aid wound toilet and maintain mobility of the patient.

INDICATIONS FOR THE USE OF EXTERNAL SKELETAL FIXATION

External skeletal fixation has valuable applications in the treatment of both acute trauma and elective surgery.

1. Some closed comminuted fractures where the fragments are large enough to take transfixing pins, and traction is not suitable.

2. Fractures associated with extensive damage to the soft tissues where traction is not suitable, and where the frequent application of dressings or skin grafting is required, or a vascular reconstruction or nerve suture needs protection.

3. Fractures with significant loss of bone, such as following gunshot injuries, where it is essential to maintain the length of the limb.

4. Multiple fractures, to allow the treatment of other fractures by traction.

5. Pelvic fractures with disruption of the symphysis pubis.

6. Arthrodesis where immobilisation in a cast is not adequate and internal fixation is not desirable.

7. Lengthening of a limb. Progressive daily distraction is possible.

8. Plastic surgical procedures, such as cross-leg flap grafts where temporary reliable fixation of the limbs is needed.

9. Failure of union following a fracture or osteotomy, especially if the overlying skin is unhealthy.

10. Infected fractures.

CONTRA-INDICATIONS TO THE USE OF EXTERNAL SKELETAL FIXATION

1. Very soft osteoporotic bone.
2. Where the bony fragments are too small to securely accept sufficient pins.
3. Infected lesions at the sites where the pins would have to be inserted.
4. Situations where it would be impossible to keep the patient under regular supervision.
5. When the surgeon is not familiar with the equipment or the method of application.

CHOICE OF EXTERNAL SKELETAL FIXATION SYSTEM

Unfortunately it is not yet known with what degree of rigidity a fractured bone should be held to obtain optimal union.

Union of a fracture occurs by a series of processes, each of which is controlled in a different way by environmental factors (McKibbin, 1978). Initially there is a short-lived primary callus response, which appears to be a fundamental reaction of bone to injury and which does not seem to be influenced by either movement or total rigidity at the fracture site. Following this initial response, is the phase in which bridging external callus is formed. This phase, which also will not continue indefinitely, is rapid, appears to depend upon the recruitment of cells from the surrounding tissues, and may be suppressed by rigid immobilisation of the fracture. If bridging of the fracture is achieved, remodelling will occur in association with a further phase of late medullary callus formation. This process is slow and appears to be assisted by immobilisation. If a fracture is treated by rigid internal fixation, the formation of external bridging callus is suppressed (Anderson, 1965) and union occurs by the formation of medullary callus and primary bone union.

Sarmiento and Latta (1981) found that external bridging callus did not form satisfactorily in response to the functional bracing of tibial fractures unless the brace was applied within six weeks of the fracture occurring.

Hicks (1977) however has shown that to obtain bony union in cases of delayed union and non-union of the hypertrophic type, more rigid fixation is required.

The choice of which system of external skeletal fixation to use depends upon the type available and the complexity and site of the bony and soft tissue injury. Generally the simpler the injury to be treated, the simpler the system can be. What is important is that if the system used initially is very rigid, then this rigidity must be decreased later to encourage bony union, perhaps being replaced by a functional cast brace.

Most systems are designed primarily for use in the management of fractures of the tibia, but some are more versatile and can be used in the management of fractures of the femur, pelvis and upper limbs. Recently, what have been termed mini systems have been introduced for use with fractures of the clavicle, metacarpals, phalanges and metatarsals. It is very important that the challenge of the application of an external skeletal fixation system to a fracture is not allowed to obscure the possibility that a safer and simpler method of treating that fracture may exist.

Described below are three of the large variety of external skeletal fixation systems which are available commercially.

Portsmouth external fixation bar (Denham external fixation compression*)

This device (Fig. 16.2), designed primarily for use in the management of complicated fractures of the tibia (Edge and Denham, 1979, 1981) consists of a single threaded steel bar. Self-tapping half-pins with continuous thread are inserted into previously drilled holes in the subcutaneous antero-medial surface of the tibia, three above and three below the fracture. The pins are fixed to carriages on the bar by acrylic bone cement (two packets to each carriage). One of the carriages is mobile, its position on the bar being governed by locking nuts. The pins in each group at either end of the bar do not have to be parallel. The two groups of pins can be distracted or approximated but cannot be angulated or rotated relative to each other once the cement has hardened. It is therefore very

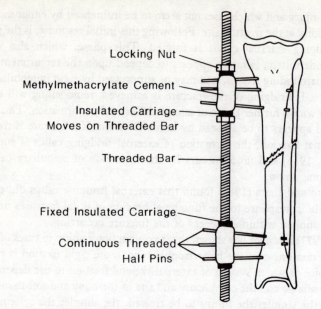

Fig. 16.2 Portsmouth external fixation bar (Denham external fixation compression).

important to try and obtain, by open operation if necessary, as accurate a reduction of the bony fragments as possible, before cementing the pins to the carriages. Obtaining a good reduction is helped by cementing only one group of pins at a time. Compression is then applied by tightening the appropriate locking nut.

A further development of this system utilizes a bar in which there is a lockable universal joint (Fig. 16.3). This enables the position of the bony fragments to be adjusted after the acrylic cement has hardened.

Universal Day frame*

This system (Fig. 16.4) also is designed for use in the management of fractures of the tibia. Two or more transfixing pins are driven through the bone and soft tissues above and below the fracture site. The pins in each group are parallel. Clamps are attached to both ends of each group of transfixing pins. Two horizontal bars, one on each side of the limb, are attached to the clamps by universal joints. This system allows adjustment of the position of the fracture in all three planes. Compression or distraction can be applied.

Hoffmann external fixation system*

The Hoffman external fixation system (Fig. 16.5) is very versatile. Half-pins or transfixing pins, either alone or in combination, can be used, but the pins in each group must be parallel. Each major component of the frame can be adjusted in

*See Appendix.

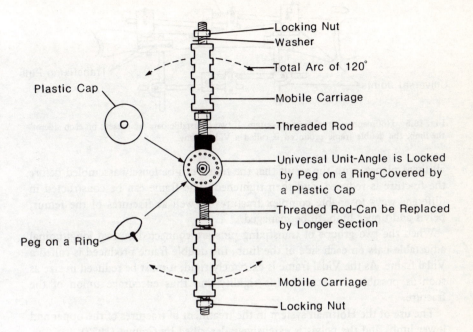

Fig. 16.3 Portsmouth external fixation bar, Mark II.

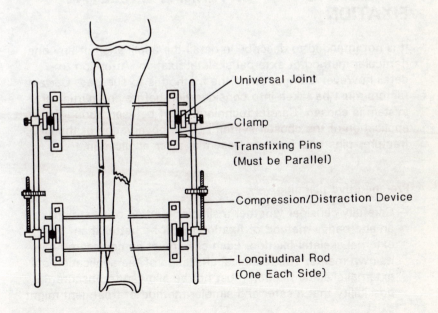

Fig. 16.4 Universal Day frame.

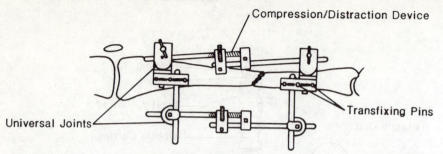

Fig. 16.5 Hoffmann external fixation system. If two adjustable bars are present on each side of the limb, the double frame produced is called a Vidal frame.

all three planes, with the result that the frame can be loosely assembled before the fracture is reduced, and then tightened. The frame can be constructed in different ways to enable complex fractures as well as fractures of the femur, pelvis and upper limb, to be managed.

When the two groups of transfixing pins are connected by two longitudinal adjustable bars on each side of the limb, the double frame produced is called a Vidal frame. As the Vidal frame is extremely rigid, it must be reduced in size as soon as possible to decrease this rigidity and thus encourage union of the fracture.

The use of the Hoffman system in the treatment of fractures of the upper and lower limbs and the pelvis is extensively described by Connes (1977).

APPLICATION OF EXTERNAL SKELETAL FIXATION

It is not intended to describe in detail the application of any one particular method of external skeletal fixation. Attention to detail however is important if the method is to succeed. Certain factors must be taken into consideration before any particular system is chosen. Careful technique must be used during the application of the chosen system. Close observation of the limb, fracture, pins and frame is essential after application.

Pre-operative planning

— Carefully consider whether a simpler method of treatment or an alternative method of fixation might be better than external skeletal fixation. Each case must be considered on its own merits. The technical challenge of the application of external skeletal fixation must not be allowed to obscure the possibility that a safer and simpler method of treatment might exist.

— Obtain good quality radiographs to enable an accurate assessment of the extent of the fracture to be made. In particular to ensure that there is not a fracture line at the intended site of insertion of the pins.
— Consider and choose the type of pins and frame most suitable for the fracture.
— Choose the best sites for insertion of the pins, taking into account the bony fragments, and ease of access for any soft tissue procedures which might be needed.
— Have a trial run with the apparatus, if possible, to check that all the necessary components are present, and that the planned frame will work as intended.

Points about technique

— Take full aseptic precautions. If iodine is used for preparation of the skin, take care that it is not left on the stainless steel pins or frame as it will cause corrosion.
— Carry out any wound cleaning which might be needed, and if possible reduce the fracture and hold the reduction with bone clamps while the pins are being inserted and the frame constructed.
— Make adequate stab wounds before inserting the pins. With self-drilling and self-tapping pins, tap the end of the pins so that their sharp points dig into the bone. This will prevent them from slipping when drilling begins. With half-pins with a continuous thread, the bone must be drilled first. With half-pins with interrupted thread, check their length radiographically before insertion.
— Use a hand brace to drill the pins into the bone. With a power drill there is a greater danger of thermal necrosis of the bone and subsequent loosening of the pin and perhaps infection of the pin track.
— Advance the pins until the threaded portions of the pins engage both cortices of the bone. If a pin is to transfix the whole limb, the skin must be incised where the pin emerges to avoid skin tension and perhaps necrosis.
— If it is essential that all the pins in one group are parallel, then a jig must be used to insert the second and all subsequent pins in any group.
— Depending upon the system chosen, either reduce the fracture and secure the pins to the frame with acrylic bone cement (Portsmouth External Fixation Bar), or connect clamps to the groups of pins then build the rest of the frame and adjust it until radiographs show that the bony fragments are in the desired position.

— Apply compression across the fracture site if the configuration of the fracture will allow it. Compression will promote union (Dwyer, 1973).

— If a limb is being lengthened, the pins and frame must be secure before the bone is divided. Distraction can then proceed without risk of deformity.

— Dress the pin sites and check that all the clamps and nuts are tight.

— Cover the sharp ends of the transfixing pins with plastic or metal caps.

Post-operative care

The limb and the apparatus must be examined *daily*.

— Check that the skin around the pins is neither inflamed nor under tension. The latter can cause skin necrosis and infection. With limb lengthening or a major change in the position of a fracture, the skin may have to be incised and resutured, under local anaesthesia, at the entry and exit sites of the pins.

— All clamps and nuts must be tight. A proper fitting spanner must be available.

— The sharp tips of the transfixing pins must be covered at all times, to prevent damage to the other limbs and the nursing staff.

— Any pins which become loose or infected must be removed promptly.

— The position of the bony fragments must be checked regularly with radiographs, and their position altered as necessary by adjusting the frame where this is possible.

— Attach suspension cords to the frame, so that the affected limb is elevated. This will help to reduce swelling and will also avoid the tissues of the calf, for example, being pressed against the pins.

— If external skeletal fixation is used for fractures of the tibia, attach some form of sling or drop-foot platform to the frame to prevent the development of a fixed equinus deformity of the ankle joint. Rubber shock cord luggage straps are useful for this.

— On the day after application of the device, encourage the patient to start exercising all the joints of the affected limb as much as possible.

— Keep the patient on bed rest until any skin wounds have healed, after which mobilisation non weight-bearing with crutches can begin.

— When radiographs show the presence of callus, partial weight-bearing can be allowed.

— When it appears that the fracture may be united radiographically, loosen the frame and check the condition of union clinically.

— Advise partial weight-bearing for the first 1–2 weeks after removal of the external fixation device.

COMPLICATIONS OF EXTERNAL SKELETAL FIXATION

1. **Infection of skin wounds.** This is more likely to occur if the initial incision in the skin before the insertion of the pins, was too small, or puckering of the skin around a pin has occurred.
2. **Infection of bone.** This can occur either from loosening of the pins, or failure to obtain rigid fixation of the bony fragments in an open fracture.
3. **Development of joint stiffness.** This is most likely to occur at the ankle joint, especially if transfixing pins are used in the lower end of the tibia. Clawing of the toes and stiffness of the fingers can occur after transmetatarsal or transmetacarpal location of pins.
4. **Damage to blood vessels, nerves or tendons by transfixing pins.**

REFERENCES

Abbott, L.C. (1927) The operative lengthening of the tibia and fibula. *Journal of Bone and Joint Surgery,* **9,** 128.

Anderson, L.D. (1965) Compression plate fixation and the effect of different types of internal fixation on fracture healing. *Journal of Bone and Joint Surgery,* **47-A,** 191.

Connes, H. (1977) *The Hoffmann's External Fixation: Techniques, Indications and Results,* 2nd English edn. Paris: Gead.

Dwyer, N.StJ.P. (1973) Preliminary report upon a new fixation device for fractures of long bones. *Injury,* **5,** 141.

Edge, A.J. & Denham, R.A. (1979) The Portsmouth method of external fixation of complicated tibial fractures. *Injury,* **11,** 13.

Edge, A.J. & Denham, R.A. (1981) External fixation for complicated tibial fractures. *Journal of Bone and Joint Surgery,* **63-B,** 92.

Hicks, J.H. (1970) Sepsis in Fractures. In London, P.S. (ed) *Modern Trends in Accident Surgery and Medicine,* p. 220. London: Butterworth.

Hicks, J.H. (1977) Rigid fixation as a treatment for hypertrophic non-union. *Injury,* **8,** 199.

Hoffmann, R. (1938) Du danger des fixateurs externes et des moyens d'y a pallier. *Acta Chirurge Belge,* **49,** 585.

McKibbin, B. (1978) The biology of fracture healing in long bones. *Journal of Bone and Joint Surgery,* **60-B,** 150.

Sarmiento, A. & Latta, L.L. (1981) *Closed Functional Treatment of Fractures.* Berlin: Springer-Verlag.

17.

Walking aids

Walking aids are used to increase the mobility of a patient, as they enable some of the body weight to be supported by the upper limbs. There are many different walking aids — parallel bars, walking frames, crutches and sticks — and many different types within each broad group. The correct selection of a walking aid for a particular patient is very important and depends upon:

1. Stability of the patient.
2. Strength of the patient's upper and lower limbs.
3. Degree of coordination of movement of the upper and lower limbs.
4. Degree of relief from weight-bearing required.

These aids may be sufficient in themselves or they may have to be used in conjunction with calipers or other orthopaedic appliances.

As the condition of the patient improves he may progress through the different types of walking aids. Whether or not the ultimate aim of walking unaided is achieved will depend upon the degree of any permanent residual disability.

After a prolonged illness, many patients are generally weak. This can be minimised by good nutrition and a well planned progressive course of exercises. When a walking aid is used, part of the body weight is taken by the muscles of the shoulder girdles and upper limbs. Attention may have to be paid to the strength of these muscles when planning the rehabilitation of the patient. The particular muscles used are:

1. Flexors of the fingers and thumb to hold the handgrips firmly.
2. Dorsiflexors of the wrist to stabilise the wrist in dorsiflexion, thereby obtaining the best functional position for powerful finger flexion.
3. Extensors of the elbow to stabilise the elbow in slight flexion when the body weight is taken through the upper limb.
4. Flexors of the shoulder to move the walking aid forward.
5. Depressors of the shoulder girdle to support the body weight.

To regain confidence in walking takes time. When walking is commenced it is therefore important to eliminate the fear of falling and to avoid too rapid progression.

PARALLEL BARS

Parallel bars are rigid and do not have to be moved by the patient. This enables the patient to concentrate entirely on moving his lower limbs correctly. For this reason parallel bars are often used when the patient is not stable, or initially to develop a particular pattern of gait, the patient being taught the correct sequence of arm and lower limb movement.

A full-length mirror should be placed at one end of the parallel bars. In it the patient can observe his movements and thus avoid looking at his feet, a common mistake made when any type of walking aid is used initially. A mirror is particularly helpful if the patient has lost proprioception.

Adjustment. Some parallel bars are not adjustable. If they are, adjust the distance between the bars and the height of the bars so that when they are held by the patient his elbows are in 30 degrees of flexion.

WALKING-FRAMES

A patient is not usually given a walking-frame unless he will never be able to walk with walking-sticks, tripods or crutches, as the pattern of gait acquired in a walking-frame is difficult to change. Moreover, a patient who uses a walking-frame is usually confined to his home, and is unable to manage stairs. If parallel bars are not available, however, a walking-frame is very useful initially when a patient is unstable and fearful of falling.

There are three main types of walking-frame: the standard walking-frame, the reciprocal walking-frame and the rollator. The first two are usually used for elderly patients who lack confidence in walking and are unsteady. Walking with full or partial weight bearing is possible. The rollator is usually reserved for patients suffering from neurological conditions, such as disseminated sclerosis, with incoordination of the lower limbs.

Standard walking-frame

The standard walking-frame (Fig. 17.1) is light, rigid, stable and easy to use. It consists of four almost vertical aluminium alloy tubes arranged in a rectangle, and joined together on three sides by upper and lower horizontal tubes. One long

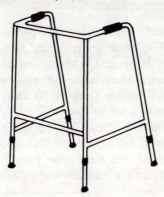

Fig. 17.1 Standard walking-frame.

side of the rectangle is left open. The lower ends of the vertical tubes, which may be adjustable by means of spring-loaded double ball catches, are fitted with rubber tips. Hand-grips are fitted to the short, upper, horizontal tubes on each side.

Adjustment. If the frame is adjustable, alter the height of *all* the vertical tubes, and ensure that they are all of equal length, so that when the handgrips are held by the patient, the patient's elbows are in 30 degrees of flexion. Patients with incoordination of the lower limbs may find walking easier if the handgrips are higher.

How to use. The patient stands in the walking-frame, lifts and places the frame forward a short distance and then walks up to the frame still holding the handgrips.

Gutter frame (forearm walker)*

The main structure of the gutter frame (Fig. 17.2) is the same as that of the standard walking frame except that the top is modified by the addition of two

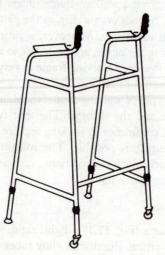

Fig. 17.2 Gutter frame.

gutters in which the patient's forearms rest. The patient takes most of his weight through the forearms. The hands grasp vertical handles to lift and turn the frame. The forearms may be secured in the gutters with light Velcro straps.

This type of frame is useful when the patient cannot extend his elbows fully or is unable to take his full weight through his hands because of weakness, deformity or the presence of a plaster cast.

The patient must be able to abduct his shoulders to 30 degrees with the forearms parallel to the floor, and must have sufficient dexterity to be able to slip one hand out of its strap and release the other forearm.

Adjustment. Adjust as for the standard walking-frame.

---

*See Appendix.

Pulpit frame (Atlas adjustable standing aid)*

The pulpit frame (Fig. 17.3) has limited application. It has the same basic shape as the standard walking frame, but it is wider and higher. The top of the frame consists of a padded U-shaped ledge which reaches the height of the lower part of the chest. The patient lifts the frame a short distance forward and then leans on the padded ledge while stepping forwards.

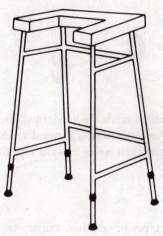

Fig. 17.3 Pulpit frame.

It is used by patients with deformity or weakness of the whole upper limb; with weak trunk muscles or ataxia; for standing practice by those who are unable to walk; and for those who tend to fall backwards when trying to walk with an ordinary walking frame, as it encourages forward flexion of the trunk.

Adjustment. Adjust as for the standard walking-frame.

Reciprocal walking-frame

A reciprocal walking-frame is basically identical with a standard frame, except that each side of the frame can be moved forward alternately. There are swivel joints between the front horizontal and vertical tubes. As the frame does not have to be lifted clear of the ground with each step, the patient's stability is increased.

Adjustment. Adjust as for the standard walking-frame.

How to use. A four-point gait is used (see Ch. 18). One side of the frame is lifted and moved forward, the two legs of the other side remaining in contact with the ground.

Rollator

A rollator (Fig. 17.4) has two small wheels at the front and two short legs at the back, protected by rubber tips. The rear legs are almost vertically under the handgrips. Care must be taken when recommending a rollator for elderly patients as it may roll too far forward so that they lose their balance.

Adjustment. Adjust as for the standard walking-frame.

*See Appendix.

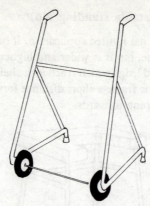

Fig. 17.4 Rollator.

How to use. The patient holds the handgrips, lifts them to raise the rear legs just off the ground, wheels the rollator forward a short distance, lowers the rear legs onto the ground and then walks forward into the rollator still holding the handgrips.

CRUTCHES

There are three main types of crutches, axillary or underarm crutches, elbow crutches and gutter crutches.

Axillary crutches

The common axillary crutches (Fig. 17.5) are made of wood. They consist of a double upright joined at the top by a padded axillary portion, a handgrip, and a non-slip rubber tip covering the lower end. The overall length of the crutch and

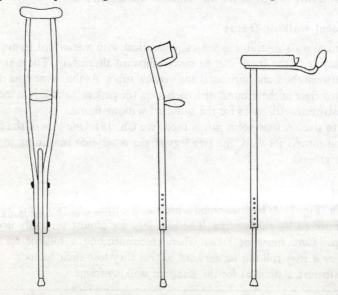

Fig. 17.5 Axillary, elbow and gutter crutches.

the position of the hand-grip should be adjustable. By using adjustable crutches, it is easier to fit each individual patient correctly, and the possible waste of cutting nonadjustable crutches to the correct size, is avoided.

When triceps weakness is present, support can be provided by attaching to the outer side of the crutch, above the level of the handgrip, a half-loop band between the double upright through which the upper arm is placed, or a short metal gutter piece to the posterior upright against which the upper arm is pressed backwards.

All degrees of weight relief are possible with axillary crutches. Usually they are used when crutch walking is commenced initially and when non-weight bearing on one lower limb is indicated, for example after a fracture. Although more cumbersome than elbow crutches, they are more stable. The patient can release a handgrip and use that hand to open a door or adjust his clothing, while continuing to support himself. This is important when the patient's balance is poor.

METHODS OF INITIAL MEASUREMENT OF LENGTH FOR AXILLARY CRUTCHES

It is necessary to be able to obtain some initial indication of the overall length of the crutches required by a particular patient. This measurement should be as accurate as possible. Final adjustment of the crutches for overall length and position of the handgrip, however, must be carried out with the patient standing and wearing shoes.

There are many methods of obtaining such a measurement. Beckwith (1965) states that the following two methods of measuring patients for axillary crutches are the most accurate.

1. Subtract 16 inches (41.0 cm) from the height of the patient, or
2. With the patient lying supine, measure the distance from the anterior axillary fold to the bottom edge of the heel of the shoe.

The measurement obtained with these two methods equals the overall length of the crutch from the top of the axillary pad to the bottom of the rubber tip.

ADJUSTMENT OF AXILLARY CRUTCHES

The overall length and the position of the handgrip must be correct for each patient.

When walking with crutches, patients wear shoes and the height of the heel will vary from patient to patient. With the patient standing up straight, the axillary crutches extend from a point 2 inches (5.0 cm) or three finger breadths below the anterior axillary fold, to a point on the ground 6 inches (15.0 cm) in front of and lateral to the tips of the toes. The shoulders are depressed and the palms of the hands rest on top of the handgrips with the elbows in 30 degrees of flexion (see Crutch Stance, Ch. 18).

Adjustment must be carried out with the patient standing and wearing shoes.
— Place a crutch under each arm.
— Check that the palms of the hands are on top of the handgrips.
— Place the tips of the crutches on the ground 6 inches (15.0 cm) in front of and lateral to the tips of the toes.
— Ask the patient to stand up straight and to relax his shoulders.

Checking overall length
— Attempt to insert three fingers between the axillary pad and the anterior axillary fold.
Too long — Less than three fingers can be inserted between the axillary pad and the anterior axillary fold. The crutches are forced into the axilla, the shoulders are hunched and the patient is unable to lift his body off the ground. Pressure on the nerves in the axilla may cause paralysis.
Too short — More than three fingers can be inserted between the axillary pad and the anterior axillary fold. The patient leans forward from the waist, his buttocks project backwards and the line of his centre of gravity passes down in front of his feet. This position is potentially unstable. It could be corrected and the pelvis brought forward by maintaining some degree of hip and knee flexion. This must not be done as it is tiring and may hinder crutch walking.

To adjust the length of the crutch
— Take off the bottom two wing nuts and remove the bolts.
— Slide the crutch extension to the correct length.
— Replace the bolts and wing nuts, but do not tighten the wing nuts at this stage, otherwise it will be impossible to move the handgrip.
— Check the overall length of the crutch again.

Checking the position of the handgrip
With the shoulder depressed and the palm of the hand on top of the handgrip, the elbow should be in 30 degrees of flexion.
Too high — The elbows are flexed more than 30 degrees, the shoulders are hunched and the ability to grip the axillary pad between the upper arm and the side wall of the chest is lost.
Too low — The palms of the hands do not rest on top of the handgrips, the axillary pad presses into the axilla, the elbows are flexed less than 30 degrees and the ability to take weight on the hands is lost.

To adjust the position of the handgrip
— Remove the uppermost wing nut and bolt.
— Move the handgrip to the correct position.
— Replace the bolt and wing nut.
— Check that the elbow is in 30 degrees of flexion.
— *Tighten all the wing nuts.*
  Note: The axillary pad must be gripped between the upper
  arm and the side wall of the chest. The patient must not lean
  on the axillary pad otherwise paralysis may occur from
  pressure of the axillary pad on the nerves in the axilla.

Elbow crutches (Loftstrand crutches)

Most elbow crutches are made from a single adjustable tube of aluminium alloy
to which are attached a U-shaped metal cuff (armband), to accommodate the
forearm just below the elbow, and a rubber or plastic covered handgrip. The
lower end is protected by a rubber tip (Fig. 17.5).

The armband is made usually from spring steel. It grips the forearm, thus
enabling the crutch to be controlled when freedom of hand movement is
required. The armband may have a front or side opening and may be fixed
rigidly or be attached by a hinge joint to the upper end of the crutch. Armbands
which are not made from spring steel and are rigidly fixed to the upper end of the
crutch can be obtained also. Occasionally for young children the armband is
replaced by a padded ring.

Adjustment of the length of the crutch between the lower end and the
handgrip is by means of a spring-loaded double-ball catch, and this mechanism is
also used in some crutches to vary the distance between the handgrip and the
armband.

Heavy duty elbow crutches, made from stainless steel tubing, are available,
and are to be preferred for those patients who for several weeks can only take
weight through one lower limb.

Elbow crutches are less cumbersome, and confer less stability than axillary
crutches, but are more stable than walking-sticks. They are prescribed for
patients who can take some weight on both feet but require an aid for balance
and confidence, for example when partial weight bearing with the three-point
crutch gait, the four-point crutch gait or the two-point crutch gait (see Chapter
18). Some patients with paraplegia, who have unusual skill, strength,
coordination and balance, may be able to use elbow crutches with the swing-
through gait.

ADJUSTMENT OF ELBOW CRUTCHES

Elbow crutches must be accurately adjusted for each patient.
Adjustment must be carried out with the patient standing and
wearing shoes.

When elbow crutches are adjusted correctly the tips of the
crutches are on the ground 6 inches (15.0 cm) in front of and

lateral to the tips of the toes and the patient is standing up straight, with his shoulders depressed and his elbows in 30 degrees of flexion.
— Ask the patient to put his arms through the armbands and to grasp the handgrips.
— Check that the palms of the hands are on top of the handgrips.
— Place the tips of the crutches on the ground, 6 inches (15.0 cm) in front of and lateral to the tips ot the toes.
— Ask the patient to stand up straight and to relax his shoulders.

Checking overall length
Too long — The shoulder is hunched and the elbow is flexed more than 30 degrees.
Too short — The patient is leaning forwards and the elbow is flexed less than 30 degrees.

To adjust the length of the crutch
— Disengage the spring-loaded double-ball catch by pressing in both buttons.
— Slightly twist the lower part of the crutch so that about half of each button is visible.
— Slide the lower part of the crutch to the desired position.
— Twist back the lower part of the crutch to allow both buttons of the ball catch to jump out.
— Check that the lower part of the crutch is firmly locked in the new position.
— Check the overall length of the crutch again.

Checking the position of the armband
The position of the armband is correct when the gap between the top of the armband and the flexor crease of the elbow is 2 inches (5.0 cm).
Adjust the position of the armband if this is possible.

Gutter crutches

A gutter crutch (Fig. 17.5) consists of a single adjustable tube of aluminium alloy. Attached to the upper end is a short horizontal metal gutter or trough in which the forearm rests with the elbow in 90 degrees of flexion. Projecting forward from the gutter is an adjustable bar carrying a vertical handgrip. The gutter, which may be padded, is secured to the forearm by Velcro fastenings. On some crutches the angle between the gutter and the alloy tube and the position of rotation of the handgrip in relation to the gutter, may be adjusted. The lower end of the crutch is protected by a rubber tip. Adjustment of length is by means of a spring-loaded double-ball catch.

Gutter crutches are indicated when there is a fixed flexion deformity of the elbow joint, weakness of the muscles controlling the elbow joint or hand, a deformity of the hand causing difficulty in gripping, or when the patient experiences pain in the hand or wrist on taking weight through the upper limb.

ADJUSTMENT OF GUTTER CRUTCHES

— Strap the forearm into the gutter so that the point of the elbow lies at or just behind the posterior edge of the gutter.
— Adjust the distance between the front of the gutter and the handgrip, so that the handgrip can be grasped firmly. If rotatory adjustment of the handgrip in relation to the gutter is possible, adjust.
— Ask the patient to stand up as straight as possible.
— Place the tip of the crutch on the ground 6 inches (15.0 cm) in front of and lateral to the tips of the toes.
— Adjust the height of the crutch by means of the spring-loaded double-ball catch so that the elbow is in 90 degrees of flexion. If the patient is unable to flex his elbow to 90 degrees, then a crutch in which the angle between the gutter and the crutch can be adjusted is required.

WALKING-STICKS

The commonly used walking-stick is made of wood, with a C-curved handle; a right-angled or pistol-grip handle is also available and may be preferred by the patient. A rubber tip protects the lower end. Adjustable sticks made from aluminium alloy tubing with rubber or moulded plastic handgrips can be obtained.

Walking-sticks are not as stable as elbow crutches, but are lighter and more easily stored. They assist balance and provide moderate support for a lower limb, and thus can improve gait and help to relieve pain, for example from a painful hip. Walking-sticks are not used unless the disabled lower limb can bear weight.

CHOOSING THE CORRECT WALKING-STICK

A patient when using a walking-stick should have his elbows in 30 degrees of flexion.

Too long — The shoulder is elevated, the elbow is flexed more than 30 degrees, ulnar deviation of the wrist is increased unless the grip on the handle is changed and support is decreased.

Too short — The patient leans forward and the elbow is flexed less than 30 degrees.

ADJUSTMENT OF WALKING-STICKS

- Place the handle of the walking-stick on the ground beside the heel of the patient's shoe.
- Remove the rubber tip.
- Adjust the length of the walking-stick so that its (lower) end is level with the most prominent part of the greater trochanter or radial styloid process.
- Replace the rubber tip.
- Reverse the walking-stick and check that the patient's elbow is in 30 degrees of flexion.

TRIPOD AND QUADRUPED WALKING AIDS

These walking aids are similar. They are made from aluminium alloy or steel tubing.

Tripod walking aid (Fig. 17.6)

This has three rubber-tipped legs which touch the ground at the corners of an equilateral triangle. The looped or right-angled handgrip lies in the same plane as a line joining two of the legs. The height of the handgrip can be adjusted.

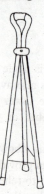

Fig. 17.6 Tripod walking aid.

Quadruped walking aid

This has four rubber-tipped legs. The handgrip lies vertically above the two inner legs, which are more widely spaced than the two outer legs. The height of the handgrip is adjustable.

The tripod and quadruped walking aids, which may be used singly or in pairs, confer more stability than walking-sticks or elbow crutches. They cannot pivot forwards and must be lifted and placed in a forward position. This requires more strength in the upper limbs than would be required for walking-sticks or crutches. Usually they are reserved for patients suffering from neurological conditions, but they may be used in the rehabilitation of elderly patients who have sustained injury to their lower limbs. These walking aids have one particular advantage over walking-sticks and crutches; they will stand upright beside a bed or a chair, ready for use.

ADJUSTMENT OF TRIPOD OR QUADRUPED WALKING AIDS

— Place the walking aid beside the patient, and ask him to take hold of the handgrip.
— Check that the aid is correctly orientated. *The handgrip must lie vertically above the two legs which are nearest to and parallel to the patient's foot* (Fig. 17.7). If the aid is positioned incorrectly, the patient will trip over the legs of the aid which lie, or will come to lie with use, in front of the patient's foot.

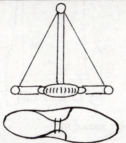

Fig. 17.7   Correct orientation of tripod walking aid. Note that the handgrip must lie vertically above the two legs of the walking aid which are nearest to and parallel to the patient's foot.

— Check that the palm of the hand lies on top of the handgrip.
— Check that the handgrip is at the correct height.
   Too high — the patient's elbow is flexed more than 30 degrees.
   Too low — the patient's elbow is flexed less than 30 degrees.

To adjust the height of the handgrip
— Loosen the adjusting screw or disengage the spring-loaded double-ball catch.
— Raise or lower the handgrip to the correct level.
— Tighten the adjusting screw or ensure that the two buttons of the ball catch are engaged.
— Check that the handgrip lies parallel to the line joining the two inner legs.
— Push down *yourself* on the handgrip to ensure that the aid will not collapse.
— Check again that the handgrip is at the correct height.

HANDGRIPS

The handgrips of all walking aids can be modified to accommodate a stiff or deformed hand. The girth of a handgrip can be increased by wrapping lengths of orthopaedic felt or sponge rubber around it. For a deformed hand, such as may occur in rheumatoid arthritis, a mould of the grip of that hand can be taken in Plastazote* and later be transferred to the handgrip of the appliance.

RUBBER TIPS

The suction-type tip is best for crutches (Fig. 17.8). It is flexible and the sides of the tip flare out slightly. There are concentric rubber rings on the undersurface,

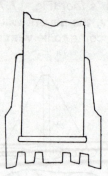

Fig. 17.8   Cross-section of a rubber suction tip.

with the outermost ring projecting slightly beyond the other rings. On a wet surface these concentric rings exert a suction-cup effect. The flexibility of the tip and the suction-cup effect ensure that the undersurface of the tip comes into uniform contact with the ground even when the walking-stick or crutch is inclined at a slight angle from the vertical.

Worn tips are dangerous. They are likely to slip. They must be replaced.

REFERENCES

Beckwith, J.M. (1965) Analysis of methods of teaching axillary crutch measurement. *Journal of the American Physical Therapy Association*, **45**, 1060.

*See Appendix.

18.

Crutch walking

The function of crutches is to prevent weight-bearing (Perkins, 1970). The majority of patients approach crutch walking with some apprehension, and the older and the more disabled the patient, the greater the apprehension. Sometimes crutches are needed only temporarily; at other times their need is permanent. The patient's ability to use crutches efficiently and perhaps eventually to walk unaided depends upon a number of factors.

1. The strength of the muscles required in the use of crutches (see Ch. 17).
2. The correct selection and adjustment of the crutches (see Ch. 17).
3. A good sense of balance.
4. Familiarity with the crutches and their maintenance.
5. The correct crutch stance.
6. Instruction in how to stand and balance with crutches before taking any steps.
7. The pattern of gait employed.
8. The energy necessary for the pattern of gait employed.
9. The initial development of the gait pattern between parallel bars if necessary.
10. Instruction and practice in walking and the performance of various manoeuvres essential for daily living, with the crutches.

CRUTCH MAINTENANCE

1. The wood or metal must not be cracked.
2. All the adjusting nuts must be tight, and all the spring-loaded double-ball catches must be working.
3. The rubber tips must be in good condition. If the tip is badly worn it must be replaced.
4. The handgrips and axillary pads if present, must be in good condition.

CRUTCH STANCE — AXILLARY CRUTCHES

Before taking any steps with the crutches, the patient must be instructed in how to stand and balance with them. This is achieved by standing the patient against a wall and placing a crutch under each arm. The correct stance with crutches is in a position with the head up, the back straight with the pelvis over the feet as much as possible, the shoulders depressed not hunched, the axillary pads of the crutches gripped between the upper arms and the side walls of the chest 2 inches (5.0 cm) below the anterior axillary fold, the crutch tips 6 inches (15.0 cm) forward and 6 inches (15.0 cm) out from the tips of the toes, the palms of the hands on top of the handgrips, the body weight taken mainly on the hands, and the elbows in a position of 30 degrees of flexion.

The correct crutch stance with elbow or gutter crutches is basically the same.

CRUTCH WALKING — PATTERNS OF GAIT

There are four different patterns of gait:

1. Swinging crutch gaits.
2. Four-point crutch gait.
3. Two-point crutch gait.
4. Three-point crutch gait.

The patterns of gait employed with crutches differ in the combination of crutch and foot or crutches and feet movements used in taking steps, and in the sequence of such combinations.

To select the pattern of gait to be employed by a particular patient, the following must be evaluated — the ability of the patient to step forward with either one or both feet; to bear weight and keep his balance on one or both lower limbs; to push his body off the ground by pressing down on both crutches; to maintain his body erect; to control the crutches; and the increased expenditure of energy required with all assisted gaits.

The two-point and the three point partial weight-bearing gaits using crutches (either axillary or elbow) or walking sticks, require 33% more energy than normal walking, whereas about 78% more energy is required by the three-point non-weight bearing and swing-through gaits (McBeath et al, 1974).

The pattern of gait which is selected should be as near normal as possible, consistent with the patient's condition. It is important to remember that walking aids are used to increase the patient's mobility. Each patient must be encouraged to walk even if he does not use a recognised pattern of gait. Any mobility is better than immobility.

It is impossible to teach any definite pattern of crutch walking to children under the age of five years. Children over the age of five can be taught but when they are alone they may not practise what they have been taught.

A distance of 12 inches (30.0 cm) is advocated as the length of step and of forward movement of the crutches when the sequence of movement in the different types of gait is described. This distance is advocated in order to emphasise that these forward movements are small and equal. It is recognised that the length of step will vary with the height of the patient. It is important that any patient who is learning to use crutches should gain confidence as quickly as possible. Confidence will be gained more quickly if the initial steps are small. As confidence increases, the length of step can be increased. When the ground is wet or slippery, short steps are advisable as slipping will be less likely to occur.

SWINGING CRUTCH GAITS

There are two types of swinging crutch gait, the swing-to crutch gait and the swing-through crutch gait. These gaits are used when the body weight can be taken through both lower limbs together but the patient is incapable of moving his lower limbs individually due to paralysis. Calipers are frequently worn to stabilise the lower limbs. The lower limbs are moved by the trunk muscles acting on the pelvis.

The stable position is that of a tripod, with a large triangular base and the apex at the shoulders. The two anterior legs of the tripod are formed by the backward and inward slanting crutches. The posterior leg of the tripod is formed by the trunk and lower limbs of the patient as he leans forward on the crutches. A patient, paralysed below the waist, is stable in this position provided that flexion contractures of the hip, knee, or ankle joints are not present, the knees are braced in extension and the centre of gravity falls in front of the hip joints, to maintain them passively in extension. If the centre of gravity falls behind the hip joints, passive hip extension will be lost, the hips will flex and the patient will collapse. Before attempting to progress the patient must practise standing in this position until he has acquired a sufficiently good sense of balance to give him confidence.

In the swing-to crutch gait, the patient advances the crutches and then swings his body to the crutches. In the swing-through crutch gait the body is swung through beyond the crutches.

SWING-TO CRUTCH GAIT

Crutch-foot sequence

Both crutches; lift and swing the body to the crutches.

The patient is in the stable position
- Place both crutches forward together a short distance.
- Take all the body weight on the hands and at the same time straighten the elbows to lift the body.
- Swing both lower limbs forward together *to between the crutches*, arching the spine as the heels touch the ground first.
- Keep the spine arched and the hips well forward. This will maintain tbe hips and knees in extension and stabilise the lower limbs.

— Take the body weight on both feet.
— *Immediately* place both crutches forward a distance of 12 inches (30.0 cm) *in front of the feet*, to regain the stable position.
— Repeat the above.

Initially, patients may not have either the confidence or the power in the upper limbs or trunk to perform the swing-to crutch gait as described above. When this occurs, the patient is taught to hitch the crutches forward and then to slide, jerk or drag the feet forward together by a body movement, while bearing down on the hand-grips and keeping the body inclined forward sufficiently to maintain the centre of gravity in front of the hip joints. As confidence and strength improve, the swing-to crutch gait will develop.

SWING-THROUGH CRUTCH GAIT

The swing-through crutch gait, although quicker than the swing-to crutch gait, must be attempted only when the patient's balance is excellent.

Crutch-foot sequence

Both crutches; lift and swing the body beyond the crutches.

The patient is in the stable position
— Place both crutches forward together a short distance.
— Take all the body weight on the hands and at the same time straighten the elbows to lift the body.
— Swing both lower limbs forward together *through the crutches*, arching the spine as the heels touch the ground first, 12 inches (30.0 cm) *in front of the crutches*.
— Keep the spine arched and the hips well forward.
— Take the body weight on both feet. The forward momentum brings the trunk and the crutches to the erect position.
— *Immediately* place both crutches forward a distance of 12 inches (30.0 cm) *in front of the feet*, to regain the stable position.
— Repeat the above.

FOUR-POINT CRUTCH GAIT

The four-point crutch gait is used when all or part of the body weight can be taken on each foot, but the patient is unsteady and therefore requires a wide base of support. As the patient's balance improves, he may progress to the two-point crutch gait.

Crutch-foot sequence

Right crutch; left foot; left crutch; right foot.

The patient is standing on BOTH feet with a crutch under each arm
— Place the *left crutch* forward a distance of 12 inches (30.0 cm).
— Step forward 12 inches (30.0 cm) with the *right foot*, taking part of the body weight on the left hand.
— Place the *right crutch* forward a distance of 12 inches (30.0 cm) *in front of the left crutch*.
— Step forward with the *left foot*, placing it 12 inches (30.0 cm) *in front of the right foot*, taking part of the body weight on the right hand.
— Repeat the above.

TWO-POINT CRUTCH GAIT

When the two-point crutch gait is used the amount of body weight taken on both feet is reduced. This type of gait is used when the patient's balance is good, some body weight can be taken through both lower limbs but both lower limbs are painful or weak.

Crutch-foot sequence

Right crutch and left foot simultaneously; left crutch and right foot simultaneously.

The patient is standing on BOTH feet with a crutch under each arm
— Place the *right crutch* and the *left foot* forward together a distance of 12 inches (30.0 cm), taking part of the body weight on the left foot.
— Place the *left crutch* and the *right foot* forward together a distance of 12 inches (30.0 cm) *in front of the left foot*, taking part of the body weight on the right foot.
— Repeat the above.

THREE-POINT CRUTCH GAIT

By using the three-point crutch gait, the amount of body weight taken by a foot can vary from none to partial or full. The three-point crutch gait is commonly taught to orthopaedic patients who may have one painful or weak lower limb which cannot support the whole body weight, and one lower limb which can. Both crutches support the weaker lower limb, while the stronger limb takes the whole body weight without any support from the crutches.

The sequence of movement of the crutches and the lower limbs in performing different functions is described below.

Crutch-foot sequence

Both crutches and the weaker lower limb together; the stronger lower limb.

WALKING, NON-WEIGHT BEARING

The patient is standing on his RIGHT foot with a crutch under each arm: the LEFT foot is off the ground.

— Take all the body weight on the *right* foot.
— Place *both* crutches forward together a distance of 12 inches (30.0 cm).
— Carry the *left* lower limb forward to a position between the crutches with the left foot off the ground. As confidence increases both crutches and the left lower limb can be advanced together.
— Take the body weight on the hands and at the same time carry the pelvis forward to between the crutches. By this means the centre of gravity passes downwards through a line between the two crutches.
— Carry the *right* foot forward and place it on the ground 12 inches (30.0 cm) *in front of* the crutches. Do not fall forwards.
— Take all the body weight on the *right* foot.
— Repeat the above.

By carrying the pelvis forward to a position between the crutches before the right foot leaves the ground, a more stable position is obtained as the pendular movement of the pelvis and lower limb is reduced and excess forward swing is avoided.

When non-weight bearing in an above-knee plaster cast, it may be necessary to add a raise to the opposite shoe, especially if the knee is held extended, to ensure that the injured limb will clear the ground as it is brought forward. If a raise is not added, the injured limb will have to be carried in front of the body with the hip in slight flexion. To ensure non-weight bearing in young children it is essential to add a raise to the opposite shoe.

When a lower limb is strong enough to take part of the body weight, that limb is placed on the ground *at the same time as the two crutches*. By this means part of the body weight is taken on the hands, and part through the lower limb. This is termed partial weight bearing.

GETTING UP FROM A CHAIR

Crutches; weak LEFT lower limb.

— Bring the heel of the *right* foot backwards to lie under the edge of the chair.
— Slide forwards on the chair so that the buttocks are resting on the edge of the chair.

— With the *right* hand, grip the arm of the chair as far forward as possible.
— Take hold of the handgrips of *both* crutches with the *left* hand.
— Place both crutches vertically on the floor near the front edge of the chair.
— Stand up by pushing upwards with the *right* leg and both arms, keeping the left foot off the ground.
— Transfer one crutch to the right hand.
— Place the crutches under the arms.
— Pause before walking to ensure that balance has been obtained.

When getting up from a wheelchair, check that the wheels are locked.

SITTING DOWN IN A CHAIR

Crutches; weak LEFT lower limb.
— After reaching the chair, check that the chair is stable. This particularly applies to wheelchairs.
— Turn round so that the *back* of the *right* leg touches the front of the chair. This aids balance.
— Take the crutches from under the arms.
— Transfer the *right* crutch to the left hand.
— Hold *both* crutches in the *left* hand.
— Place the *right hand* on the arm of the chair.
— Bend forward slightly.
— Gently lower the body onto the chair.

STEPPING UP A KERB OR STEP

The method described here is used also when going up stairs using two crutches.

Always step up with the stronger lower limb first. Crutches; weak LEFT lower limb.
— Approach the kerb.
— Place the ends of *both* crutches in the angle formed by the kerb and the road.
— Take the body weight on the hands, straighten the elbows and carry the pelvis forward to between the crutches.
— Lift the *right* foot off the ground and carry it upwards and forwards onto the kerb.
— Straighten the right knee, thereby transferring the body weight on to the right foot.
— Lift *both* crutches up and carry them and the left lower limb forwards in preparation for the next step.

STEPPING DOWN A KERB OR STEP

The following method is used also when going down stairs using two crutches.

Always step down with the crutches and the weaker lower limb together first. Crutches; weak LEFT lower limb.
— Approach the edge of the kerb.
— Take all the body weight on the *right* foot.
— Place *both* crutches downwards and 12 inches (30.0 cm) forward on the road, bending the right knee and carrying the left lower limb forward at the same time. The higher the kerb, the greater the distance the crutches must be placed away from the kerb.
— Take the body weight on both hands and carry the pelvis forward to between the crutches.
— Lift the right foot off the ground and place it downwards and forwards on the road *in front of the crutches*, thus proceeding to the next step.

ASCENDING STAIRS WITH A HANDRAIL

Crutches; weak LEFT lower limb; handrail on the RIGHT.
— Approach the bottom of the stairs.
— Transfer the *right crutch* to the left hand. It is more convenient if the *transferred* crutch is carried horizontally in the left hand.
— Take a forward grip on the handrail with the *right* hand.
— Without moving the *left* crutch, lift the body upwards and forwards with both hands and at the same time lift the *right* foot upwards and forwards onto the first step.
— Lift the left crutch up on to the *same* step.
— Repeat the procedure until the top of the stairs is reached.
— Transfer the second crutch back under the right arm before proceeding.

If the handrail is on the left, the procedure is identical except that the left crutch is transferred to the right hand. Always step up with the stronger lower limb first.

DESCENDING STAIRS WITH A HANDRAIL

Crutches; weak LEFT lower limb; handrail on the RIGHT.
— Approach the top of the stairs.
— Transfer the *right crutch* to the left hand, holding the transferred crutch horizontally.

- Place the *right* hand slightly forward on the handrail.
- Place the left crutch on the step below, bringing the left lower limb forward at the same time.
- Bend the *right knee* to bring the pelvis forward between the crutch and the right hand.
- Take the body weight on the hands.
- Lift the right foot off the ground and place it forwards and downwards on the same step as the left crutch.
- Repeat the procedure until the bottom of the stairs is reached.
- Transfer the second crutch back under the right arm before proceeding.

If the handrail is on the left, the procedure is identical except that the left crutch is transferred to the right hand. Always step down with the crutch and the weaker lower limb first.

Before a patient can be considered to be really efficient with crutches, he must be able to step backwards, forwards and sideways, and to walk on uneven surfaces and up and down inclines.

WALKING-STICKS

Walking-sticks can be used to decrease the amount of body weight taken through a lower limb during walking and therefore can compensate for muscle weakness and relieve pain. In addition the use of a walking-stick or sticks can increase the stability and the confidence of a patient.

Once a lower limb is strong enough to be able to take nearly all the body weight, two sticks can be substituted for crutches. The technique of walking with two sticks is the same as that described above for partial weight bearing with crutches. It is preferable to use two walking-sticks initially. If only one walking-stick is used, the patient will tend to lean towards the stick, to take a shorter stride on that side and to carry the opposite lower limb in abduction. This abnormal gait tends to persist after the walking-stick is abandoned. When a good technique using two walking-sticks has been achieved, one stick can be discarded. The single walking-stick is carried in the opposite hand to the affected lower limb. (Some patients, however, with a lesion of the knee or ankle, may gain more relief by holding the walking-stick in the ipsilateral hand.) For example, to obtain partial relief from weight bearing on the left foot, hold the walking-stick in the right hand, and place the left foot and the walking-stick forwards together at the same time.

Increased stability and further relief from weight bearing can be obtained by bringing the hand inward to rest against the body in the region of the greater trochanter of the femur.

REFERENCES

McBeath, A.A., Bahrke, M. & Balke, B. (1974) Efficiency of assisted ambulation determined by oxygen consumption measurement. *Journal of Bone and Joint Surgery*, **56-A**, 994.

Perkins, G. (1970) *The Ruminations of an Orthopaedic Surgeon*, p. 45. London: Butterworths.

19.

Tourniquets

In many orthopaedic operations on the upper and lower limbs, a bloodless field is important as it aids the recognition of tissues, and eliminates delay and trauma caused by repeated swabbing.

To provide a bloodless field, blood must be removed from the limb and then prevented from re-entering it. Elevation of the limb, and the reflex vasoconstriction which follows this, decreases the volume of blood within it, but more complete exsanguination can be achieved by actively squeezing the blood out of the limb. An Esmarch bandage is commonly used for this (see below). External pressure is applied at the root of the limb by a tourniquet, to occlude the arteries and veins and thereby prevent re-entry of blood.

THE DEVELOPMENT OF TOURNIQUETS

For centuries, a tightly constricting device has been applied around limbs to stop haemorrhage, especially during amputation.

The term 'tourniquet' was coined by Petit in 1718, to describe the action of his screw device (Fig. 19.1) to stop haemorrhage (Klenerman, 1962), but Lister was

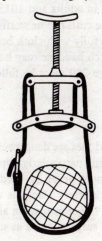

Fig. 19.1 Petit type of tourniquet.

the first surgeon to employ it to provide a bloodless field for an operation other than amputation; the excision and arthrodesis of a tuberculous wrist joint (Lister, 1909). However, he drained the limb of blood by elevation.

In 1873, Johann von Esmarch, Professor of Surgery at Kiel and Surgeon General to the army, described the bandage which bears his name. It was flat and woven from indiarubber. He used it to exsanguinate the limb, but prevented blood from re-entering by applying, around the limb, heavy rubber tubing fastened by a hook and brass chain. The Esmarch bandage later came to be used as a tourniquet as well as for exsanguination. Such use however, was associated with nerve palsies. To try to prevent these palsies occurring, Harvey Cushing, in 1904, invented the pneumatic tourniquet, developing it from the standard Riva-Rocci blood pressure apparatus. He described its use for craniotomies, but soon it was used for operations on limbs.

The pneumatic cuff is the basis for all modern tourniquets.

TYPES OF TOURNIQUET

There are two main types of tourniquet, non-pneumatic and pneumatic. The later may be non-automatic or automatic, when there is a regulating mechanism to compensate for small leaks in the system.

NON-PNEUMATIC

It is permissible only in exceptional circumstances to use a non-pneumatic tourniquet on an upper or lower limb. The danger with non-pneumatic tourniquets, whether straps or rubber bandage, is that the pressure exerted by them on the underlying tissues is unknown. Middleton and Varian (1974) have shown that with an Esmarch bandage, there is a linear increase in pressure with each turn of the bandage, with the result that the pressures under the bandage can reach 900 mm of mercury in adults and 1015 mm mercury in children.

Only a few modern pneumatic cuffs can be sterilised. An Esmarch bandage can be autoclaved if it is rolled carefully with cloth between each layer. It is thus in sterile situations that an Esmarch bandage may have to be used as a tourniquet. The procedure detailed on page 280 must be followed very carefully.

Digital tourniquets

Tourniquets around fingers and toes are dangerous, as they may not be removed at the end of the operation. This particularly applies to finger cots and silastic rings (Smellie, 1962) which must never be used. The risk of using a digital tourniquet is reduced if a large artery clamp is used to secure a large rubber catheter around the base of the finger or toe. An alternative safe tourniquet for a finger can be fashioned from a surgical glove as suggested by Karev (1979) (see below).

PNEUMATIC TOURNIQUETS

The pneumatic cuffs used as tourniquets are based on the same physical principles as blood pressure cuffs but they are stronger, their fastenings are more secure and they usually have a stiff backing piece to maintain the effective width of the inflated cuff.

Non-automatic

A non-automatic pneumatic tourniquet consists of a pneumatic cuff, a hand-operated pump and a pressure gauge. The pressure in the cuff is known but there is no automatic compensation for leaks in the system, and a regular check therefore must be kept on the pressure in the cuff. In addition the hand pump is small and it may be difficult to rapidly raise the pressure above the patient's systolic blood pressure. This could result in venous engorgement if an Esmarch bandage is not used for exsanguination.

Automatic

In an automatic pneumatic tourniquet, there is a constant supply of gas to compensate for any leaks in the system. In addition as some form of gas reservoir is used, the patient is less likely to be moved from the operating table with the tourniquet in place. A pumped reservoir may be used, but in the newer systems the gas comes from a container of a very volatile liquid (dichloro-difluoro-methane), from bottled air or nitrogen, or from the compressed air line to the operating theatre.

With any of the above systems, the inflation of the cuff is rapid and controllable thus essentially eliminating the chance of venous engorgement occurring.

CONTRA-INDICATIONS TO EXPRESSIVE EXSANGUINATION

1. **Severe infections and tumour.** When either of these two conditions are present, expressive exsanguination must not be used, to avoid dissemination.
2. **Proven or suspected deep vein thrombosis.** When proven or suspected deep vein thrombosis is present expressive exsanguination must not be used. Austin (1963) reported two cases in which massive fatal pulmonary embolism was precipitated by exsanguination with an Esmarch bandage in the presence of silent deep vein thrombosis. Both patients had sustained fractures around the ankle, initially treated by manipulation and immobilisation in a plaster cast, which 7 to 9 days later required internal fixation.

CONTRA-INDICATIONS TO THE USE OF A TOURNIQUET

1. **Peripheral arterial disease.**
2. **Severe crushing injuries.** In these cases the circulation is often precarious.
3. **Sickle-cell disease.** Under anoxic conditions the red blood corpuscles sickle, blood viscosity increases, vessels become blocked and a severe episode of thrombosis and haemolysis may occur, particularly on release of the tourniquet. *Test all patients who are at risk* for the presence of Haemoglobin–S prior to the use of a tourniquet.

SITE FOR APPLICATION OF A TOURNIQUET

With the exception of digital tourniquets, it is now accepted that tourniquets must only be placed around the upper arm or thigh. These are the only places where there is sufficient muscle bulk to distribute the pressure in the cuff evenly, and thus avoid local high pressure areas over tissues close to the surface. Cuffs must not be placed around the forearm, wrist or ankle.

WIDTH OF PNEUMATIC CUFFS

The American Heart Association concluded that for the pressure in the occluding cuff of a sphygmomanometer to equal that in an underlying central artery, the width of the cuff should be 20% greater than the diameter of the upper arm, and be 40% of the circumference of the thigh or 8 inches (20 cm). If cuffs of these dimensions can be used, the pressures in them need only be a little above the systolic blood pressure, to maintain a bloodless field. If narrower cuffs have to be used, higher pressures are needed to transmit sufficient pressure to the centre of the limb to occlude the artery. Tissues immediately beneath a cuff may be submitted to possibly excessive and damaging pressure. To avoid this therefore, the widest practicable cuff, up to the dimensions given above, must always be used.

EXSANGUINATION

The simplest and safest way to remove most of the blood from a limb, is to elevate the limb as vertically as possible for four minutes. Blood drains from the veins under the effect of gravity, and this is followed by reflex arteriolar constriction which makes the emptying more complete. More efficient exsanguination can be achieved by inflating an envelope covering the whole limb (Klenerman, 1978), or by applying an Esmarch bandage from the digits to the cuff (see below).

TOURNIQUET PRESSURES

It is important that the pressure in a cuff is known accurately at all times. Cushing's simple and reliable method was to connect the cuff to the mercury manometer of an ordinary sphygmomanometer. Although this method is still in use, most systems now use a dial gauge as this is more convenient and can read higher pressures than an ordinary blood pressure mercury column. These dial gauges, which must record pressure in mm of mercury, are simple to use, but can become inaccurate with damage or long use (Flatt, 1972; Fry, 1972). Hallett (1982) found 14 out of 52 dial gauges in daily use to be seriously inaccurate.

Experimental work and clinical observation have shown that much lower pressures can be used than has been the custom in recent years (Klenerman and Hulands, 1979; Klenerman et al, 1980; Klenerman, 1982). The pressure to be used is based upon the unsedated patient's blood pressure measured on the ward before operation.

For the upper limb, the pressure should be 50 mm of mercury higher than the systolic blood pressure, whereas for the lower limb, it should be twice the systolic blood pressure. The higher pressure is needed for the lower limb because a cuff of the ideal width may be too wide to fit on the thigh above the operative field.

| UPPER LIMB (mm of Hg) | SYSTOLIC BLOOD PRESSURE PLUS 50 |
| LOWER LIMB (mm of Hg) | TWICE THE SYSTOLIC BLOOD PRESSURE |

TOURNIQUET TIME

Tourniquets must be applied for the shortest possible time, compatible with proper surgery. For a healthy patient a safe routine is for the surgeon to be notified after one hour and for him to remove the cuff as soon as possible after that. If the operation is difficult the time may be extended to $1\frac{1}{2}$ hours, and 2 hours probably should be regarded as the maximum. These times, however, will not be safe for all patients. Special care must be taken with the elderly, and patients suffering from diabetes and alcoholism.

Flatt (1972) set a time limit of two hours for 1500 consecutive operations on the hand and found that 95% of the operations could be completed within that time. Complications did not occur in the 60 patients whose operations exceeded that time. The two nerve palsies which occurred in the other patients were traced to faulty equipment. He stated, 'Two hours is not safe, but one hour can be exceeded if proper equipment is being used'.

Klenerman, and his fellow workers (Klenerman et al, 1980; Klenerman, 1982) have suggested, following their research on healthy monkeys and humans, that a longer period is safe as long as the minimum effective pressure is used. They agree that the longer period will not apply to patients who are unwell, or who have a manifest or subclinical neuropathy.

DANGERS OF A TOURNIQUET

Tourniquets are dangerous. It must be remembered that the advantage of using a tourniquet is mainly to the surgeon, therefore risks to the patient are not justified (Bonney, 1981).

Major complications from the use of a tourniquet are rare. Middleton and Varian (1974) estimated that the overall incidence of major complications was 1:8000, being 1:5000 in the upper limb and 1:13 000 in the lower limb. Flatt (1972) reported major complications due to faulty equipment in 2 out of 1500 operations on the upper limb. Most of the complications which occur could be avoided if all the facts now known about tourniquets are taken into account.

The dramatic complications of gangrene from an excessive period of ischaemia, and nerve palsies from excessive pressure, have been known for a long time. Experience in two World Wars has shown the risk to both life and limb which results from leaving tourniquets applied for too long under battle conditions. They should only be used as a last resort (Watson-Jones, 1952).

Most attention has been directed recently towards the dangers from pressure, with the suggestion that longer periods of ischaemia can be tolerated (Klenerman et al, 1980). This may result in other problems due to ischaemia being uncovered.

The dangers from the use of a tourniquet can result from the process of exsanguination, from pressure on the tissues under the tourniquet, from ischaemia, from bleeding after closure of the wound and from failure to remove the tourniquet after the end of the operation. Each of these will be considered separately.

DANGERS FROM EXSANGUINATION

Exsanguination by elevation is not hazardous, but there are risks when it is achieved by compression. Frictional shearing forces from a tightly applied Esmarch bandage can damage the skin, especially when it is weakened by conditions such as senility, rheumatoid arthritis, steroids or the Ehlers-Danlos syndrome. The ends of fractured bones, bone screws or foreign bodies may damage skin or soft tissues if the bandage is applied tightly. Nerves which lie subcutaneously can be damaged unless protected by additional padding.

Compressive exsanguination must not be used in the presence of deep venous thrombosis, malignant tumour or infection, all of which might be spread by embolization.

Austin (1963) reported two cases in which massive fatal pulmonary embolism was precipitated by exsanguination with an Esmarch bandage in the presence of silent deep vein thrombosis. Both patients had sustained fractures around the ankle, initially treated by manipulation and immobilization in a plaster cast, which 7 to 9 days later required internal fixation.

During an operation under a tourniquet, injury to a major blood vessel may occur and not be recognised. Patrick (1963) described four cases of injury to the popliteal artery which occurred during operations for the removal of menisci. None of the injuries was recognised at the time of the operation.

Blockage of the superficial femoral artery from disruption of an atheromatous plaque, in a young woman, has also been reported (Giannestras et al, 1977).

The heart may be overloaded, with possible cardiac arrest, if both lower limbs are exsanguinated at the same time in an elderly or unfit patient. Effective exsanguination of both lower limbs will result in 15% of the circulating blood volume being forced back into the remaining circulation. This equals a rapid transfusion of 700–800 ml of blood (Klenerman, 1982). This extra cardiac load can be tolerated by the young healthy patient. In the elderly or unfit patient, a tourniquet should be applied to only one limb at a time.

DANGERS FROM THE PRESSURE IN THE TOURNIQUET CUFF

Most tourniquet cuffs need a layer of wool or foam padding under them to protect the skin from pinching and abrasion as the cuff is inflated. Care must be taken to ensure that irritant or inflammable skin preparation solutions do not soak under the cuff. Skin necrosis has been recorded (Flatt, 1972; Middleton & Varian, 1974), but not ignition from diathermy. This complication can be prevented by covering the cuff and the adjacent skin with an adherent plastic drape.

Occasionally the walls of arteries are stiffened by calcium deposits and the rigid tubes that result cannot be compressed by normal cuff pressures (Klenerman, 1976). If the pressure is increased there is a risk that the vessel walls will fracture and that the blood supply to the limb will be damaged permanently. Urgent surgical exploration of the artery could be required.

Even without an unusually high pressure in the cuff, local damage under the cuff can occur if the skin is fragile, the bone irregular or the normal padding from muscle and fat is absent, for example in cachexia, severe rheumatoid arthritis and poliomyelitis. In these situations, extra padding under the cuff must be used.

If the pressure in the cuff is higher than necessary, normal skin, muscles and nerves are at risk. Muscle is the tissue most likely to suffer permanent damage, but the most severe functional disability results from damage to nerves. Healthy nerves are more resistant than muscle to structural damage from pressure, but the function of nerves is impaired rapidly by both pressure and ischaemia (Lewis et al, 1931).

When a nerve sustains local injury from pressure, the effect is seen over the whole area distal to the site of injury, supplied by that nerve. The effect of injury to a muscle is restricted to that muscle and its action.

Unhealthy nerves such as those in patients suffering from diabetes mellitus, alcoholism and rheumatoid arthritis are at greater risk than normal.

The effect of pressure on muscle has been studied by Patterson and Klenerman (1979) in healthy monkeys. Damage was more marked under the cuff than distally. Mitochondrial changes were seen at one hour and increased to their maximum at five hours. After up to three hours of compression, recovery was rapid and the muscle had a normal histological appearance when examined 24 hours later. Muscle power took a week to return to normal. After five hours of compression there was extensive mitochondrial damage and necrotic fibres were seen three days later.

Tourniquet paralysis syndrome

The tourniquet paralysis syndrome is caused by pressure rather than ischaemia. It was described by Moldaver in 1954 as having the following features.

1. Motor paralysis with hypotonia or atonia but without appreciable atrophy.
2. Sensory dissociation. Touch, pressure, vibration and position sense usually are absent, as these modalities are carried by large fibres which are more sensitive to pressure. Pain sensibility rarely is lost and hyperalgesia may be present. The recognition of heat and cold usually is preserved.
3. The colour and temperature of the skin are normal as sympathetic function is not affected.
4. The peripheral pulses are normal.

Electrical studies show that the block to nerve conduction is at the level of the tourniquet. Motor nerve stimulation distal to the block may still produce a contraction. Pressure distorts the myelin sheaths which retract from the nodes of Ranvier. This process continues as segmental demyelination. The axons are preserved (Ochoa et al, 1972). The pathological condition of tourniquet paralysis syndrome is probably an extension of the physiological state of rapidly recoverable paralysis which occurs when the pressure in a blood pressure cuff has been held above the systolic blood pressure, in an unanaesthetised subject, for about half an hour (Bonney, 1981). Recovery from full paralysis takes three months (Moldaver, 1954; Middleton and Varian, 1974).

DANGERS FROM ISCHAEMIA

The tissues distal to the cuff become anoxic, acidotic and loaded with metabolites (Wilgis, 1971; Klenerman et al, 1980). Wilgis felt that critical levels of acidosis were reached after two hours, as the venous pH in the limb had fallen to 6.90, the pO_2 had fallen to 4 mm Hg and the pCO_2 had risen to 104 mm Hg. Klenerman et al (1980) did not measure the pO_2 but found that the pH levels did not fall so low in either monkeys or humans. They found that after three hours of ischaemia it took 40 minutes for the acid-base levels in the limb to return to normal. With ischaemia of more than three hours duration the recovery time increased dramatically. They do not feel that there is any benefit in the practice, advocated by Bruner (1951), of releasing the tourniquet for ten minutes after one hour to allow the limb to recover, during the course of an operation which will take over $1\frac{1}{2}$ or 2 hours. They base their opinion on their finding that the return to normal takes 20 minutes after one hour, and that the capillary bed is not perfused for the first few minutes after the release of the tourniquet (Wilgis, 1971). Wilgis also found that arteriolar shunting resulted in poor initial oxygen uptake. We feel that the practice of briefly releasing the tourniquet should not simply be abandoned because the limb is unable to return completely to normal in the time allowed, as such practice may result in the limb being better able to withstand a further period of ischaemia. The matter remains controversial.

Tourniquets and sickle cell disease

The use of a tourniquet is almost certainly contra-indicated in *sickle cell disease*. The blood in a limb will sickle if a tourniquet is used. However, in patients with *sickle cell trait*, doctors who work in Africa and the West Indies have not reported any particular problems with tourniquets (Klenerman, 1982). If a tourniquet must be used in a patient with *sickle cell trait*, the limb must be exsanguinated thoroughly before the cuff is inflated, and the period of ischaemia must be kept to an absolute minimum.

Post-tourniquet syndrome

Following the release of a tourniquet there is immediate swelling of the tissues, due partly to reactive hyperaemia and partly to increased capillary permeability to fluids and protein. Klenerman (1982) found that the swelling became much more severe when the tourniquet time was increased beyond two hours. If this swelling is severe and is allowed to persist, the condition merges into the post-tourniquet syndrome.

The post-tourniquet syndrome is probably due to ischaemia and its duration. Certainly the longer the period of ischaemia and the older the patient, the more likely it is that untoward tissue reactions will occur. Bruner (1951) described the post-tourniquet syndrome in the upper limb as consisting of the following:

1. Puffiness of the hand and fingers, evidenced by a smoothing out of the normal skin creases.
2. Stiffness of the joints in the hand to a degree not otherwise explained.
3. Colour changes in the hand which is pale when elevated and congested when dependent.
4. Subjective sensations of numbness without true anaesthesia.
5. Objective evidence of weakness of the muscles in the hand and forearm without real paralysis.

PREVENTION OF THE POST-TOURNIQUET SYNDROME

To decrease the degree of congestion of the tissues and to minimise haematoma formation at the operative site:

— **Select the correct operation for each patient.** As the tissues of elderly patients are less tolerant of ischaemia, swelling and stiffness are more likely to occur after operation. To carry out a lengthy operation may result therefore in a decrease rather than an increase in function.

— **Avoid wasting time.** It is imperative that the duration of tissue ischaemia is kept to a minimum. As already stated this is achieved by:

Careful pre-operative planning of the operation to avoid wasteful movements.

Delaying the application of the tourniquet until all necessary instruments are ready, the surgeon is scrubbed, gowned and ready to cleanse the skin, the patient is on the operating table and the operating lights are adjusted.

— **Do not extend the tourniquet time unnecessarily.** It is better to suture tendons after the tourniquet has been released rather than to prolong the duration of tissue ischaemia. Nerves must always be sutured and skin grafts applied after release of the tourniquet to avoid the formation of a haematoma between the nerve ends or under the skin graft.

— **Ensure good haemostasis.** If the tourniquet is released before the wound is closed, capillary haemorrhage is controlled by local pressure with saline compresses for 5 to 10 minutes, after which the larger vessels are clamped and ligated. If the wound is closed, a bulky dressing under moderate compression by a crepe bandage must be applied before the tourniquet is released.

— **Elevate the limb after the operation.**

— **Encourage the patient to perform active movements** of the pertinent part.

DANGERS FROM BLEEDING AFTER CLOSURE OF THE WOUND

If a tourniquet is released before the wound is closed, any major source of haemorrhage can be identified and controlled. This may prevent the formation of a haematoma jeopardising wound healing. Generally tourniquets are released before a nerve is sutured or a skin graft applied, to ensure that a haematoma does not separate the tissues.

With some operations there is bleeding from bone which cannot be stopped until a firm dressing is applied. In these cases it is better to insert a drain and keep the cuff inflated until the dressing is secure.

It is safer to release the tourniquet before closure if there is any risk that a major blood vessel may have been damaged. Injury to the popliteal artery during meniscectomy, which was not recognised at the time of operation, has been reported (Patrick, 1963).

DANGERS FROM FAILING TO REMOVE THE TOURNIQUET

Failure to remove a tourniquet is most likely to occur with digital tourniquets, especially if rubber rings or bands without large clips are used (Chen, 1973; Hoare 1973). The patients life will not be threatened by metabolites from an ischaemic finger, so the tourniquet can always be released when it is discovered and efforts made to save the finger.

Six hours has been suggested as the dividing line between removing the cuff and trying to save the limb, and removing the limb above the cuff to save the patient's life (Klenerman, 1962). *The nursing staff must call the medical staff BEFORE removing any forgotten tourniquet.* If a tourniquet is removed, preparations must be made to treat the crush syndrome which may develop (Bywaters and Beall, 1941; Mason, 1978). It is encouraging to note that Middleton and Varian (1974) reported full recovery after a tourniquet had been left in place for $4\frac{1}{2}$ hours, although there were initial sciatic and femoral nerve palsies.

ROUTINE CHECKS ON TOURNIQUET EQUIPMENT

The surgeon must satisfy himself that the tourniquet equipment he uses is correctly maintained and that all gauges are accurate.

BEFORE EVERY OPERATING LIST

— Check the level of the fluid in the reservoir or the pressure of gas in the cylinder.
— Ensure that the machine will attain and hold a pre-set pressure. Set a pressure, block the distal end of the tubing going to the cuff, and inflate.
— Inspect the cuff, its fasteners, and all connections and tubing.

MONTHLY

— Inspect the Esmarch bandage for tears or perished areas. Ensure that tapes are attached if it is ever used as a tourniquet.
— Check the pneumatic cuff system for leaks. If the cuff is applied over a rigid cylinder, a pre-set pressure should be maintained for an hour without a drop in the level of the reservoir.
— Check that the pressure gauge on the control unit is accurate when connected to a mercury manometer, over the range covered by the mecury column (0–300 mm). Due to the simple mechanical nature of the gauges most commonly used, they are unlikely to be dangerously inaccurate if readings at 100, 200, and 300 mm Hg are all correct to within a few millimetres. Perform the test by connecting the tube, which goes to the pneumatic cuff, directly to the tube to the mercury manometer of an ordinary sphygmomanometer.
— The controls and gauges must be checked over their full range, and all seals and connections overhauled at the intervals recommended by the manufacturer, as well as after every time a fault is found.

RECORDS OF USE OF A TOURNIQUET

Records must be kept every time a tourniquet is used, so that if complications do occur, it is possible to retrieve all the information that is needed for research or medico-legal purposes. Pre-printed cards, such as illustrated below, on which all the relevant information can be recorded, should be present in the patient's case records.

Table 19.1

Tourniquet record sheet		
Date	Name	Hosp. No
		D of B
Surgeon	Address	
	Operation	
Type — Pneumatic	Cuff site — Upper Arm	
Esmarch B	Thigh	
Other	Digit	
	Other	
Method of exsanguination		
Elevation	Cuff width	
Esmarch B		
	Cuff pressure	mm Hg
Return of circulation		
Within ONE Minute	Duration On	
After Minutes	Off	
Not at all	Total	Minutes

HOW TO APPLY AN ESMARCH BANDAGE FOR EXSANGUINATION

An assistant is necessary.
— Elevate the limb.
— Wrap the Esmarch bandage around the limb, starting at the hand or foot and working proximally. The extreme tips of the fingers and toes and the heel can be left free.
— Fully stretch each turn of the bandage before applying it to the limb.
— Overlap each turn of the bandage by $\frac{1}{2}$ inch (1.25 cm).

HOW TO APPLY AN ESMARCH BANDAGE AS A TOURNIQUET

The use of an Esmarch bandage as a tourniquet is not recommended as the pressure exerted by it on the underlying tissues is unknown, and will probably be higher than is advisable. However, it is recognised that special circumstances or particular local problems may make its use as a tourniquet necessary. If this is so, then the Esmarch bandage must be applied very carefully and the tourniquet time kept to the absolute minimum.

— Apply an Esmarch bandage as described for exsanguination, but make sure that the application starts with the end of the bandage to which the tapes are attached.

— At the upper thigh or upper arm, wrap the Esmarch bandage over padding, the last 4 or 5 turns being on top of each other. *Only the first turn of the bandage is applied with tension. The last three or four turns must only be wrapped loosely around the limb.*

— Slip the remaining roll of the bandage under the last turn so that it lies in the line of the artery.

— Unwind the distal end of the bandage, starting at the fingers or toes, until the turns acting as a tourniquet are reached.

— Tie the two end tapes securely to the table to guard against the patient leaving the theatre with the tourniquet still in place.

— Note the time, and enter it on the tourniquet record sheet.

— Remember to keep the tourniquet time as short as possible.

HOW TO APPLY A DIGITAL TOURNIQUET

1. Fingers and toes

— Clean and anaesthetise the digit.

— Wrap a layer of gauze snugly around the base of the digit, to prevent the skin being pinched.

— Elevate the hand or foot for four minutes, or squeeze the digit firmly.

— Ask an assistant to wrap a single turn of rubber tubing over the gauze and to pull it tight.

— Secure the tubing with a large artery clip, in such a way that the handle of the clip is out of the way.

— Note the time and enter it on the tourniquet record sheet.

2. Fingers only (Karev, 1979)

— Clean the hand and anaesthetise the relevant finger.

— Ease a sterile surgical glove over the finger and the rest of the hand.

— Cut a small hole in the tip of the glove of the required finger.

— Roll back the glove to the base of that finger.

— Note the time and enter it on the tourniquet record sheet.

The finger is now exsanguinated and will remain so while the glove is in place. The rest of the hand has a sterile covering.

HOW TO APPLY A PNEUMATIC TOURNIQUET

An assistant is necessary.
- Apply a few layers of orthopaedic wool, or a towel, around the limb at the tourniquet site.
- Choose the correct size of pneumatic cuff (upper limb, lower limb or paediatric).
- Express all air from the pneumatic cuff.
- Snugly wrap the pneumatic cuff around the limb on top of the padding.
- Ensure that the connecting tube lies on the outer aspect of the limb, and points proximally.
- Reinforce the Velcro, or other type of fastening of the pneumatic cuff, with zinc oxide strapping or a cotton bandage.
- Elevate the limb for four minutes, or —
- Exsanguinate the limb by applying an Esmarch bandage as described above, stopping the bandage 1–2 inches (2.5–5.0 cm) below the pneumatic cuff. If the Esmarch bandage is applied up to the level of the cuff, the cuff may slip distally at the time of inflation, or the pressure in the cuff may be so lowered on removal of the Esmarch bandage that bleeding may occur during the operation.
- Raise the pressure in the cuff rapidly to the predetermined level (see above) to prevent filling of the superficial veins before the arterial blood flow has been occluded.
- Note the time and write it down.
- Remove the Esmarch bandage.

WHEN A TOURNIQUET IS USED

- Use a colourless skin preparation solution especially for the toes and fingers. The state of the circulation in the toes or fingers will be determined more easily after the operation.
- Do not allow the skin preparation solution to collect under the edge of the tourniquet. Skin irritation or burning may result. To avoid this a self-adhesive drape (Steridrape*; Opsite*) can be applied over the neighbouring skin and the tourniquet.
- If the pressure of the tourniquet should fall during the operation, remove the tourniquet completely to relieve congestion before reapplying it.

*See Appendix.

- Do not allow the tissues exposed at the operative site to become dry. Regularly apply cold saline compresses.
- Avoid the use of hot spot-lights which will accelerate the drying of the tissues.
- *At the end of the operation remove the tourniquet. This is the responsibility of the surgeon. Note the time at which the tourniquet is removed.*
- *At the end of the operation check that the circulation in the limb is satisfactory* — peripheral pulses and/or capillary circulation.

BIER'S BLOCK

Double pneumatic cuffs (Hoyle, 1964) have been introduced as an ingenious method of reducing the pain from the tourniquet cuff in regional intravenous analgesia (Bier, 1908). However a potentially serious problem exists with a double cuff, as each cuff is only half the width of the cuff which normally would be used on the arm. If the normal cuff pressure is used (see above), the veins are occluded, but the arteries are not, with resultant venous congestion. If the pressure in the cuff is increased until arterial flow ceases, tissues beneath the cuff may be damaged. It may be safer if double cuffs are not used for the Bier's technique. Pain due to pressure of the cuff is an occasional problem, but as long as the operating time is limited to less than 40 minutes, additional analgesia will rarely be required.

APPLICATION OF BIER'S BLOCK FOR THE UPPER LIMB (Ware, 1975)

This technique is absolutely contra-indicated for any patient with a known hypersensitivity to local anaesthetic solutions.

It is potentially dangerous. Five serious incidents including three deaths have been reported. It is recommended that the tourniquet equipment must be used and constantly monitored by one person who is familiar with it and whose sole duty is anaesthesia (Department of Health and Social Security, Health Notice (Hazard)(82)7).

- Lie the patient supine.
- Dilute 20 ml 0.5% PLAIN Bupivacaine Hydrochloride[†] (Marcain*, Duncan Flockhart & Co. Ltd) to a final volume of 50 ml with Sodium Chloride Injection BP solution, using a 50 ml syringe. This will produce an 0.2% solution of Bupivacaine Hydrochloride. *The maximum recommended dosage is 1.5 mg/kg body weight.*

---

*See Appendix.
[†]See Important Note (p. 285).

Table 19.2

Weight of Patient (kg)	Bupivacaine dose at 1.5 mg/kg (mg)	Final injection volume of 0.2% solution (ml)
70	105	52.5
60	90	45
50	75	37.5
40	60	30

Note: The final volume of 0.2% solution of Bupivacaine Hydrochloride is equal to half the dose in mg of Bupivacaine Hydrochloride, calculated at 1.5 mg/kg body weight.
— Measure the patient's blood pressure.
— Apply a tourniquet cuff to the upper arm, but do not inflate it.
— Insert a small (23G) indwelling needle or plastic cannula into a suitable vein, preferably on the dorsum of the hand. Secure the needle.
— Exsanguinate the limb by elevation for four minutes or by the use of an Esmarch bandage.
— Inflate the cuff to a pressure 50 mm mercury higher than the systolic blood pressure, and maintain this pressure for the duration of the operation.
— Inject the required dose of 0.2% bupivacaine, and then gently massage the limb to facilitate the spread of the anaesthetic solution. The patient will experience a feeling of warmth and/or paraesthesia.
— Wait for analgesia to develop. This usually occurs within 4 to 6 minutes. Loss of cutaneous sensation to pin prick is a useful guide. As muscle relaxation occurs the limb will feel 'heavy' to the patient. If analgesia is patchy or inadequate, inject a further 5 to 10 ml of the 0.2% bupivacaine solution.
— Note the time and enter it on the tourniquet record sheet.
— On completion of the operation, deflate the cuff and note the time for entry on the tourniquet record sheet.
— Remove the indwelling needle. Sensation will usually return within 8 minutes.
— Allow the patient to recover under supervision.

Bupivacaine Hydrochloride is recommended because of its low level of systemic toxicity (Ware and Caldwell, 1976). It is however longer acting and is approximately four times as potent as Lignocaine Hydrochloride (Xylocaine*, Astra Pharmaceuticals Ltd) which can also be used. *The maximum recommended dosage of Lignocaine Hydrochloride is 3.0 mg/kg body weight.*

Toxic reactions to local anaesthetic solutions are unpredictable, and depend

*See Appendix.

upon the dosage, route of administration and the physical state of the patient. They include nervousness, dizziness, blurred vision, nausea, vomiting, tremor, convulsions and cardiac arrest.

Adequate resuscitation equipment must be available.

IMPORTANT NOTE ON THE USE OF BUPIVACAINE

Since first publication of this edition a strong warning has been issued by the Committee on Safety of Medicines (C.S.M., 1983) that Bupivacaine (Marcaine) should no longer be used for Bier's Block. It is now felt that serious complications (including cardiac arrest) are more likely to occur than with Lignocaine and are much more resistant to treatment.

REFERENCES

Austin, M. (1963) The Esmarch bandage and pulmonary embolism. *Journal of Bone and Joint Surgery*, **45-B**, 384.
Bywaters, E.G.L. & Beall, D. (1941) Crush injuries with impairment of renal function. *British Medical Journal*, **i**, 427.
Bier, A. (1908) Ueber Einen Neuen Weg Localanästhesie An Den Gliedmassen Zu Erzeugen. *Archiv Für Klinische Chirurgie*, **86**, 1007.
Bonney, G.L.W. (1981) Personal communication.
Bruner, J.M. (1951) Safety factors in the use of the pneumatic tourniquet for haemostasis in surgery of the hand. *Journal of Bone and Joint Surgery*, **33-A**, 221.
Chen, S.C. (1973) Ring tourniquets for fingers. *British Medical Journal*, **iv**, 174.
Committee on Safety of Medicines (Oct 1983) Bupivacaine (Marcaine Plain) in intravenous regional anaesthesia (Bier's Block). *Current Problems*, **No. 12.**
Cushing, H. (1904) Pneumatic tourniquets: with especial reference to their use in craniotomies. *Medical News*, **84**, 577.
Esmarch, J.F.A. von (1873) Ueber Künstliche Blutleere bei Operationen. Sammlung Klinischer Vortäge in Verbindung mit Deutschen Klinikern. *Chirurgie*, **19, No. 58**, 373.
Flatt, A.E. (1972) Tourniquet time in hand surgery. *Archives of Surgery*, **104**, 190.
Fry, D. (1972) Inaccurate tourniquet gauges. *British Medical Journal*, **i**, 511.
Giannestras, N.J., Cranley, J.J. & Lentz, M. (1977) Occlusion of the tibial artery after a foot operation under tourniquet. A case report. *Journal of Bone and Joint Surgery*, **59-A**, 682.
Hallett, J.P. (1982) Personal communication.
Hoare, E.M. (1973) Simple finger tourniquet. *British Medical Journal*, **iii**, 293.
Hoyle, J.R. (1964) Tourniquet for intravenous regional analgesia. *Anaesthesia*, **19:2**, 294.
Karev, A. (1979) A simple finger tourniquet. *British Journal of Plastic Surgery*, **32**, 136.
Klenerman, L. (1962) The tourniquet in surgery. *Journal of Bone and Joint Surgery*, **44-B**, 937.
Klenerman, L. (1976) Incompressible vessels. *Lancet*, **i**, 811.
Klenerman, L. (1978) A modified tourniquet. *Journal Royal Society of Medicine*, **71**, 121.
Klenerman, L. & Hulands, G.H. (1979) Tourniquet pressures for the lower limb. *Journal of Bone and Joint Surgery*, **61-A**, 124.
Klenerman, L., Biswas, M., Hulands, G.H. & Rhodes, A.M. (1980) Systemic and local effects of the application of a tourniquet. *Journal of Bone and Joint Surgery*, **62-B**, 385.
Klenerman, L. (1982) Personal communication.
Lewis, T., Pickering, G. & Rothschild, P. (1931) Centripetal paralysis arising out of arrested blood flow to the limb. *Heart*, **1**, 31.
Lister, J. (1909) *Collected Papers*, Vol. 1, p. 176. Oxford: Clarenden.
Mason, J.K. (1978) *The Pathology of Violent Injury*. London: Arnold.
Middleton, R.W.D. & Varian, J.P.W. (1974) Tourniquet paralysis. *Australian and New Zealand Journal of Surgery*, **44**, 124.
Moldaver, J. (1954) Tourniquet paralysis syndrome. *American Medical Association Archives of Surgery*, **68**, 136.

Ochoa, J., Fowler, T.J. & Gilliatt, R.W. (1972) Anatomical changes in peripheral nerves compressed by pneumatic tourniquet. *Journal of Anatomy*, **113**, 433.

Patrick, J. (1963) Aneurysm of the popliteal vessels after meniscectomy. *Journal of Bone and Joint Surgery*, **45-B**, 570.

Patterson, S. & Klenerman, L. (1979) The effect of pneumatic tourniquets on the ultrastructure of skeletal muscle. *Journal of Bone and Joint Surgery*, **61-B**, 178.

Smellie, G.D. (1962) Exsanguinating finger tourniquet. *Lancet*, **ii**, 78.

Ware, R.J. (1975) Intravenous regional analgesia using Bupivacaine. *Anaesthesia*, **30**, 817.

Ware, R.J. & Caldwell, J. (1976) Clinical and pharmacological studies of intravenous regional analgesia using Bupivacaine. *British Journal of Anaesthesia*, **48**, 1124.

Watson-Jones, R. (1952) *Fractures and Joint Injuries*, Vol. 1, 4th edn, p. 121. Edinburgh: Livingstone.

Wilgis, E.F.S. (1971) Observations on the effect of tourniquet ischaemia. *Journal of Bone and Joint Surgery*, **53-A**, 1343.

Appendix 1

Ace Orthopedic
14105 South Avalon Boulevard
Los Angeles
California 90061
USA.

Ace cervical traction equipment
Halo-body orthosis
(UK distributors, see
Downs Surgical Ltd)

Apex Foot Products
New York
USA.

Dermaplast shoes

Arthrodax Ltd
Arthrodax House
Telford Road
Bicester
Oxfordshire OX6 OTZ
England.

Cellamin
Cellona

Astra Pharmaceuticals Ltd
St Peters House
2 Bricket Road
St Albans
Herts AL1 3JW
England.

Xylocaine
(Lignocaine Hydrochloride)

Bayer (UK) Ltd
Pharmaceutical Division
Haywards Heath
West Sussex RH16 1TP
England.

Baycast (in USA — Cuttercast)

Bury Boot & Shoe Co. (1953)
Ltd
Woodhill Works
Brandlesholme Road
Bury
Lancashire BL8 1BG
England.

Various styles of men's and women's
shoes in broad and extra broad
fittings

B X L Plastics Ltd   Plastazote (manufacturers)
ERP Division
Mitcham Road
Croydon
Surrey CR9 3AL
England.

Carters Ltd   Atlas adjustable frame (Pulpit frame)
Alfred Street
Westbury
Wiltshire
England.

Chas A. Blatchford & Sons Ltd Metal hinges and jig for cast bracing
Lister Road
Basingstoke
Hants RG22 4AH
England.

C & L Developments   Hadfield split bed
47 Queens Road
Weybridge
Surrey
England.

Cutter Laboratories Inc.   Cuttercast (in UK — Baycast)
2200 Powell Street
Emeryville
California 94608
USA.

D. Howse & Co. Ltd   Simonis swivel
Beethoven Street
London W10 4LR
England.

Downs Surgical Ltd   Ace cervical traction equipment —
Church Path   UK distributor
Mitcham
Surrey CR4 3UE
England.

Duncan, Flockhart & Co. Ltd Marcain (Bupivacaine Hydrochloride)
Birkbeck Street
London E2 6LA
England.

George Salter Ltd   Suspension springs for a Thomas's
West Bromwich   splint
Staffordshire
England.

Gilbert & Mellish Ltd
501–503 Bristol Road
Selly Oak
Birmingham B29 6AU
England.

Howmedica Inc.
Orthopedics Division
359 Veterans Boulevard
Rutherford
New Jersey 07070
USA.

Howmedica (UK) Ltd
622 Western Avenue
Park Royal
London W3 0TF
England.

Jaquet Orthopedie S.A.
45 Avenue de la Praille
Case Postale 380
1211 Geneve 26
Switzerland.

J. E. Hanger & Co. Ltd
Roehampton Lane
Roehampton
London SW15 5PL
England.

John Drew (London) Ltd
Orthopaedic Supplies Dept
433 Uxbridge Road
Ealing
London W5
England.

Johnson & Johnson Ltd
Orthopaedic Division
260 Bath Road
Slough
Berks SL1 4EA
England.

Johnson & Johnson Products
Ltd
New Brunswick
New Jersey 08903
USA.

Piedro bootees — UK distributor

Hoffmann external fixation system —
UK distributor
Universal Day frame

Hoffmann external fixation system

Ortholene

Drushoes

Neofract
Orthoflex
Orthoplast functional bracing kits
Specialist foam traction
Tractac
Zoroc

Delta-lite fabric
Delta-lite glass

Marlin Orthotics
177 Grange Road
London SE1
England.

Boston brace — UK distributors

Minnesota Mining
& Manufacturing Co.
Orthopedic Products
Surgical Products Division/3M
3M Centre
St Paul
Minnesota 55144
USA.

Lightcast II
Scotchcast
Scotchflex
Steridrape

United Kingdom Ltd
3M House, PO Box 1
Bracknell
Berkshire RG12 1JU
England.

Lightcast II
Scotchcast
Scotchflex
Steridrape

OEC Orthopaedic Ltd
134 Brompton Road
London SW3 1JB
England

Denham external fixation compression
(Portsmouth external fixation bar,
Mark I & II)
Orthotrac (in USA — Orth-O-Trac)
Zimmer electric plaster saw

Orthopedic Equipment Co.
Bourbon
Indiana
USA.

Orth-O-Trac

Orthopaedic Systems
40 Mersey Road
Widness
Cheshire WA8 0DS
England.

Hexcelite

Parke, Davis & Co.
Pontypool
Monmouthshire
Wales.

Ketalar (Ketamine Hydrochloride)

Performance Plastics Ltd
Melton Mowbray
Leicestershire
England.

Perplas

Physical Support Systems Inc.
Windham
New Hampshire.

Boston brace

Pryor & Howard Ltd
Willow Lane
Mitcham
Surrey
England.

Brackets for attaching Böhler stirrup to
Thomas's splint for suspension
by springs
Fisk splint

Radiol Chemicals Ltd
Stepfield
Witham
Essex CM8 3AG
England.

Soesi shoe laces

Remploy Ltd
Orthopaedic Division
415 Edgware Road
Cricklewood
London NW2 6LR
England.

Eagle bootees
Forearm walker (Gutter frame)

Salt & Son Ltd
220 Corporation Street
Birmingham
England.

Hartshill lower limb appliances

Seton Products Ltd
Tubiton House
Medlock Street
Oldham
Lancashire OL1 3HS
England.

Notac
Seton skin traction kits
Tubigrip

S. H. Camp & Co. Ltd
East Portway
Andover
Hants SP10 3NL
England.

Four poster cervical brace
Pavlik harness
Somi brace — UK distributors

Smith & Nephew Ltd
Bessemer Road
Welwyn Garden City
Hertfordshire
England.

Crystona
Elastoplast skin traction kits (outside the
British Commonwealth, all Elastoplast
products are known under the name
Tensoplast)
Glassona
Gypsona
Opsite
Plastazote — UK distributors

S. Reed & Co.
Beechwood House
Infirmary Road
Blackburn
Lancashire BB2 3LP
England.

Prefabricated tibial brace

The Scholl Manufacturing Co. Ltd
182–204 St John Street
London
England.

Ventfoam skin traction bandage

United States Manufacturing Co.
PO Box 110
623 South Central Avenue
Glendale
California 91209
USA.

Fracture bracing components

Victor Baldwin Ltd
Vansitard Estate
Windsor
Berkshire
England.

Yampi, supplied in various colours

Zimmer USA
727 North Detroit
Warsaw
Indiana 46580
USA.

Skin-trac
Pelvic traction screw
Screw eye — Wing traction screw — for olecranon traction

Zimmer Deloro Surgical Ltd
Dunbeath Road
Elgin Industrial Estate
Swindon
Wiltshire SN2 6EA
England.

Pelvic traction screw
Screw eye — Wing traction screw — for olecranon traction

Appendix 2

TECHNICAL ANALYSIS FORM   **RIGHT UPPER LIMB**

Name _____ No. _____ Age _____ Sex _____

Date of Onset _____ Cause _____

Occupation _____ Present Upper-Limb Equipment _____

Diagnosis _____

Hand Dominance: Right ☐ Left ☐

Status of other upper limb: Normal ☐   Impaired ☐

1.   Ambulatory status: Normal ☐   Impaired ☐   Walking Aid ☐

2.   Wheelchair ☐   Sitting Position: Stable ☐   Unstable ☐   Reclined ☐   Upright ☐
     Sitting Tolerance: Normal ☐   Limited ☐   Duration _____
     Propulsion: Manual ☐   Motor ☐   Dependent ☐

3.   Cognition: Normal ☐   Impaired ☐

4.   Endurance: Normal ☐   Impaired ☐

5.   Skin: Normal ☐   Impaired ☐

6.   Pain ☐   Location _____

7.   Vision: Normal ☐   Impaired ☐

8.   Coordination: Normal ☐   Impaired ☐   Function: Normal ☐   Compromised ☐
                                                            Prevented ☐

9.   Motivation: Good ☐   Fair ☐   Poor ☐

10. Associated impairments: _____

─────────────────────────────── **LEGEND** ───────────────────────────────

⊕ ↓1 = Direction of Translatory Motion *(Grade 1,2 or 3)*	**Volitional Force (V)** N = Normal G = Good F = Fair P = Poor T = Trace Z = Zero	**Sensation** N = Normal (boxed) ▦ = Hypesthesia ▨ = Paresthesia ▩ = Anesthesia
⊕ 60° = Abnormal Degree of Rotary Motion		
⊕ 30° = Fixed Position	**Hypertonic Muscle (H)** N = Normal M = Mild Mo = Moderate S = Severe	**Proprioception (P)** N = Normal I = Impaired A = Absent
⋀⋁ = Fracture		D = Distension or Enlargement

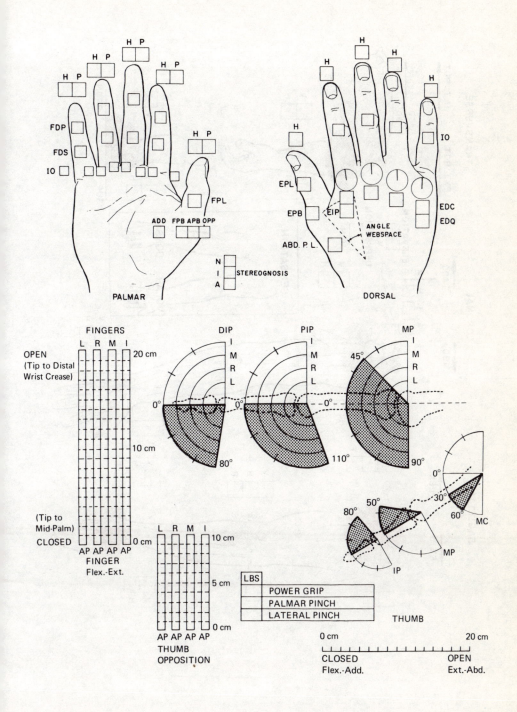

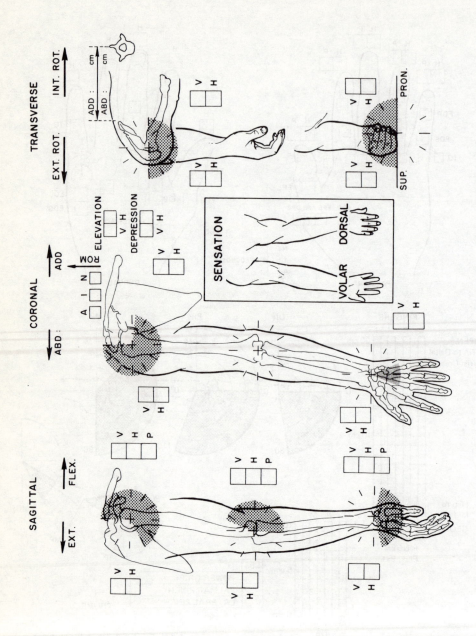

Summary of Functional Disability _____

_____

_____

_____

_____

Treatment Objectives: Prevent/Correct Deformity ☐   Improve Function ☐
                         Relieve Pain ☐   Other _____

ORTHOTIC RECOMMENDATION

UPPER LIMB		FLEX	EXT	ABD	ADD	ROTATION Int.	ROTATION Ext.	AXIAL LOAD
SEWHO	Shoulder							
EWHO	*Humerus*							
	Elbow							
	Forearm							
WHO	Wrist			(RD)	(UD)			
HO	Hand							
Fingers 2-5	MP							
	PIP							
	DIP							
Thumb	CM					(Opposition)		
	MP							
	IP							

REMARKS:

_____   _____
            Signature   Date

KEY: Use the following symbols to indicate desired control of designated function:

F = FREE   — *Free* motion.
A = ASSIST   — Application of an external force for the purpose of increasing the range, velocity, or force of a motion.
R = RESIST   — Application of an external force for the purpose of decreasing the velocity or force of a motion.
S = STOP   — Inclusion of a static unit to deter an undesired motion in one direction.
v = Variable — A unit that can be adjusted without making a structural change.
H = HOLD   — Elimination of all motion in prescribed plane (verify position).
L = LOCK   — Device includes an optional lock.

TECHNICAL ANALYSIS FORM   **SPINE**

Name_____ No._____ Age____ Sex____ Weight_____ Height _____

Diagnosis_____ Occupation _____

Present Orthotic Equipment _____

_____

Ambulatory☐   Non Ambulatory☐   Wheelchair☐

Standing Balance: Normal ☐   Impaired ☐   Walking Aid _____

Sitting Position: Stable☐   Unstable☐   Reclined ☐   Upright ☐

Sitting Tolerance: Normal☐   Limited ☐

MAJOR IMPAIRMENTS

A. Structural: No Impairment ☐

    1. Bone: Osteoporosis ☐   Fracture☐   Level_____

            Other_____

    2. Disc Space: (Describe)_____

    3. Alignment: Scoliosis☐   Kyphosis☐   Lordosis ☐

B. Sensory: No Impairment ☐

    1. Anesthesia☐   Location _____

    2. Pain☐   Location_____

C. Upper Limb: No Impairment ☐

    1. Amputation☐ _____

    2. Other_____

D. Lower Limb: No Impairment ☐

    1. Limb Shortening: Right☐   Left☐   Amount _____

    2. Hip Contracture ☐   Ankylosis☐   Flexion☐   Degree _____

        Adduction☐   Degree_____   Abduction☐   Degree _____

        Extension☐   Degree_____

    3. Major Motor Loss☐   Location _____

    4. Sensation: Anesthesia☐   Location_____

        Hypesthesia☐   Location _____

        Pain☐   Location _____

E. Associated Impairments:_____

_____

LEGEND

ARTHRODESIS

ARTHRITIS

FRACTURE

SEGMENTAL
INSTABILITY

Q = QUADRATUS
LUMBORUM

I = ILIOPSOAS

VOLITIONAL FORCE
(V)

N = NORMAL
G = GOOD
F = FAIR
P = POOR
T = TRACE
Z = ZERO

HYPERTONICITY
(H)

N = NORMAL
M = MILD
Mo = MODERATE
S = SEVERE

T5

T8 (deg.)

T12

CURVE WITH
APICAL VERTEBRA

% OF NORMAL
MOTION

%

= PELVIC
TILT

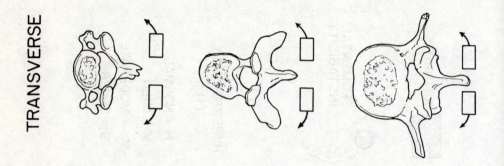

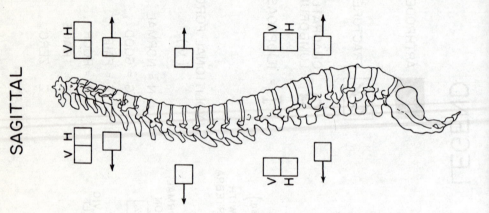

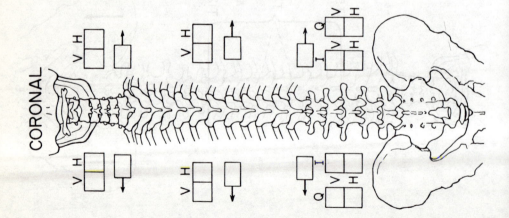

Summary of Functional Disability:_____

_____

_____

Treatment Objectives:

      Spinal Alignment ☐   Motion Control ☐

      Axial Unloading ☐   Other _____

_____

ORTHOTIC RECOMMENDATION

SPINE		FLEX	EXT	LATERAL FLEXION		ROTATION		AXIAL LOAD
				R	L	R	L	
CTLSO	Cervical							
TLSO	Thoracic							
LSO	Lumbar							
	(Lumbo sacral							
SIO	Sacroiliac	▓	▓	▓	▓	▓	▓	

REMARKS:

_____

KEY: Use the following symbols to indicate desired control of designated function:

    F = FREE   – Free motion

    A = ASSIST – Application of an external force for the purpose of increasing the range, velocity, or force of a motion.

    R = RESIST – Application of an external force for the purpose of decreasing the velocity or force of a motion.

    S = STOP   – Inclusion of a static unit to deter an undesired motion in one direction.

    v = Variable – A unit that can be adjusted without making a structural change.

    H = HOLD   – Elimination of all motion in prescribed plane: specify position, e.g. in degrees or (+) (–).

    L = LOCK   – Device includes an optional lock.

                                  Signature _____

                                      Date _____

Index